THE SNAKE IN THE CLINIC

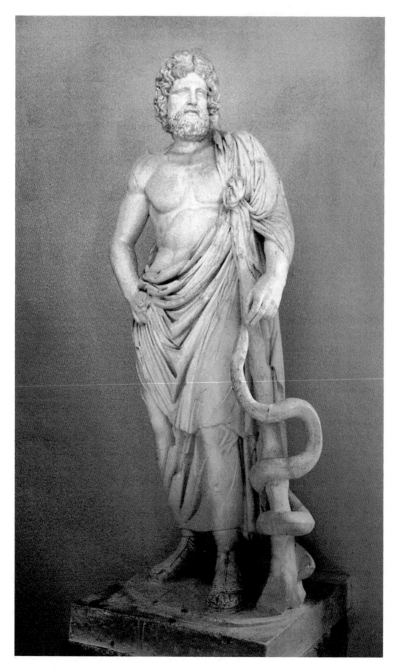

Asklepios statue at Epidaurus.

THE SNAKE IN THE CLINIC
Psychotherapy's Role in Medicine and Healing

Guy Dargert

KARNAC

First published in 2016 by
Karnac Books Ltd
118 Finchley Road
London NW3 5HT

British Library Cataloguing in Publication Data

A C.I.P. for this book is available from the British Library

ISBN-13: 978-1-78220-374-2

Typeset by V Publishing Solutions Pvt Ltd., Chennai, India

www.karnacbooks.com

Dedicated to
Asklepios

With indebtedness and thanks to
Chris Jenkins, Pippa Weitz, Rod Tweedy, Tony Bernacca,
Patrick Harpur,
and most of all to Jas Salamander
for her unfailing encouragement and support.

CONTENTS

ACKNOWLEDGEMENTS

Chapter One is composed of previously published articles. The first part of the chapter was initially published in the winter 2008 edition of the *Thresholds Journal* of the *Association for Pastoral and Spiritual Care* under the title of "Attending to psyche". Later it appeared in the United Kingdom Council for Psychotherapy (UKCP)'s magazine *The Psychotherapist* under the title "Defining psychotherapy" in issue 48, summer 2011. The second part of the chapter appeared in *The Psychotherapist* under the title "Illness is a part of health" in issue 57, summer 2014.

ABOUT THE AUTHOR

Guy Dargert is an American-born psychotherapist with thirty-five years' experience of practice who now lives and works in Cornwall. Over his career he has practised psychotherapy in a wide variety of medical and educational settings as well as in private practice. He has taught on numerous university level training courses. He is currently an Honorary Fellow of Exeter University and teaches courses in medical humanities to students at the Peninsula College of Medicine and Dentistry.

FOREWORD

Patrick Harpur

The Snake in the Clinic is a marvellous book. It should be read by all psychotherapists; but, lucidly written and free of unnecessary jargon, it would be an especially wise companion for anyone starting out in the profession. Although I was hoping for a plea on behalf of the soul's primacy (which the book undoubtedly is) I was surprised and delighted to find that the book begins by eloquently entreating us to be mindful of symptoms. Guy is only too aware of how they are commonly dealt with: his discussion of drug use—and of drugs versus placebos—is both witty and chilling. He sees in so much modern treatment the tendency to stifle symptoms instead of discerning them. But if we can bring ourselves to listen to symptoms—those forlorn, muffled cries of a soul buried beneath the rubble of our lives—then we might hear what the soul really wants and uncover the roots of our disorders.

Guy goes on to show us (his examples, drawn from his own clients, are pertinent and packed with insight) how symptoms should not be confused with illness itself but, rather, how both can be read as paths to the deeper reaches of the psyche where the cause of illness lies. In short, *The Snake in the Clinic* embodies that very perspective which it advocates, where "perspective" means a "seeing through" the symptom to the symbol beneath.

Nor is the book's depth solely one of perception—it's also historical. The fascinating chapter on the ancient Greek origins of Western medicine under the aegis of Asklepios, god of healing, argues that the psychological and the physical, mind and body, were never meant to be divorced as they now usually are. On the contrary, both were honoured in a sacred environment especially constructed to be both beautiful and cathartic in order to promote that wholeness which is cognate with healing. Indeed, psychotherapy itself is, or should be, such a temple. It has its own uniqueness and integrity. It recognises the unity or, perhaps, the co-inherence of a soul and body that have become dislocated, and creates an intermediate, imaginative space where they can be re-adjusted to each other and a greater wholeness entertained.

Following James Hillman's "acorn and oak" model of the soul's unfolding, Guy boldly asserts that all our lives have a *telos*—an aim, end or pattern which it is our task to fulfil, just as if Plato were right when he recounted in the myth of Er how we pre-natally choose a life presided over by a guiding and protective personal daimon. It's little wonder, then, that whenever we betray our life-pattern we are plagued by the daimons of physical and psychological symptoms which paradoxically signpost our path to recovery even as they point to where we have strayed.

The Snake in the Clinic is as broad-minded as it is deep, as outward-looking as it is introspective. Guy does not want us isolated in our skins or skulls. He encourages us to consider how our dis-eases may have their roots in family, in the environment, in social circumstances—that is, in the world. I particularly like his notion that the *genius loci*, the spirit of a place, may well play an unacknowledged part, for good or ill, in our personal psychology.

The more I read this book, the more I became convinced that it was not only for psychotherapists: if only members of the medical profession could be persuaded to read it as well, they might be reminded to pay closer attention to a patient's illness and so to discern beneath the apparent facts of a case history the metaphors of the soul's true story.

time that I first encountered his ideas in Fordham's book and the fact that it occurred on the anniversary of his birth.

The desire to make sense of this mystifying, wondrous, and unsettling experience led me into a lifelong fascination with the world of psychotherapy. It led me first of all into my own experience of personal psychotherapy. Eventually it took me to psychotherapy training and to the study and practice of psychoanalytic and humanistic psychotherapies including body and breath work. In the course of a very varied career as a practitioner of group and individual psychotherapy and as a supervisor of other practitioners, I have worked in cities and in rural areas, in universities, general medical practices, half way houses for the mentally ill, and in counselling agencies. I have run public groups and workshops. I have also lectured in a number of universities, been a staff mediator with the British National Health Service and a consultant lecturer in a medical college. I have had many opportunities both to practise psychotherapy and to verbally convey my understanding of what I believe is good practice to people with extraordinarily different backgrounds, assumptions, and personal issues. I have needed to draw on many different frames of reference to achieve this.

Over the three and a half decades of my practice to date I have seen the psychotherapy profession evolve. I welcome the fact that psychotherapy has become less of an elitist activity that was available in the main only to those fortunate enough to have the money to fund it. Today it has become more mainstream and democratised. However, in my view this has regrettably often been at the cost of dumbing down the profession. Ever more we seem prone to quantifying, commodifying, rationalising, and industrialising our work; work which I deeply believe is in its essence an extraordinary mystery. During this time trainings have increasingly moved into college and university settings where they have taken on an academic emphasis at the expense of experiential learning and intuitive understanding. Perhaps academia by its very nature must favour what can be objectively measured. Additionally, there are often economic pressures on trainers to fill courses with students. Under this kind of pressure candidates who are able enough to deal with the intellectual demands of training are accepted. However not all trainees may be ready, willing, or able to deal with the profound experiential and personal demands of an in-depth training. Candidates who have no prior experience of personal therapy are often accepted. At the same time many funders of psychotherapeutic care are inclined to want fast and tangible results that can be measured. I feel that the more subtle aspects of psychological development can be undervalued, overlooked, and neglected as a result of this. We can forget that psychotherapy is essentially the work of attending to the mystery of the soul in order to bring about healing.

In common with the medical world, psychotherapy has seen a trend toward developing ever greater specialisations. We have witnessed a steady stream of new medical and psychological diagnostic labels. These often come handily accompanied by new medications and psychological treatments. We seem to want to be ever greater experts in ever more specific conditions. We come to know more and more about less and less as we colonise obscure and newly discovered corners of the psychotherapy marketplace. We forget that healing is about "wholing"— the bringing together of disconnected parts of a whole with the hope and the expectation that this will help to harmonise and lessen the disease between them. We can overlook the broader picture of what it is that we are doing as psychotherapists. We need to be mindful of more than how we contribute to the healing of specific conditions that belong to specific persons. We are also a part of a much greater and broader process of healing that affects the community and society of which we are a part. The work of psychotherapy touches the soul of the world.

What I aim to do in the following pages is to draw together some of the threads that have run through my understanding of what it means to be a psychotherapist. I have drawn not just on psychological theory from a number of different schools of therapy, but also on scientific research, mythology, ethnography, spiritual traditions, and personal experiences in therapy with some of those clients who have privileged me by sharing their stories, their struggles, and their transformations. What I write of this is essentially true and illustrative of the kind of work we have done in therapy. I have fictionalised only to the point of anonymising their identity.

In what follows I invite readers to look beyond the rational, reductionist, and marketplace view of psychotherapy. I aim to draw attention to the much more expansive picture of which our work is crucial part. Our work is a contemporary permutation on an ancient and universal theme. There is reason to believe that we are rooted in and draw on timeless and global traditions of healing that give weight, substance, and relevance to our work.

CHAPTER ONE

Psychotherapy and health

Defining psychotherapy

Psychotherapy is a set of techniques used to treat mental health and emotional problems and some psychiatric disorders.

(National Health Service, 2008)

Words have a life of their own. The word "psychotherapy" for instance carries a history. It was employed in the late nineteenth century by a French medic and hypnotist named Hippolyte Bernheim who used it to distinguish his technique from that of his contemporary Jean-Martin Charcot. The spelling we use is a transliteration from the Greek of the two words that make up his chosen term. The letters represent its correct pronunciation in Greek. These two words each have a specific meaning. Just as people carry the resonance of their past, so too do words. The modern word continues subconsciously to carry these meanings. To what are we essentially referring when we use this word? When we examine the word we reach a different and a deeper understanding to that offered by the National Health Service.

Is there any historic resonance to the NHS's description of psychotherapy as a "set of techniques?" The Greek word *therapia* means to "give attention to" or "to attend to" in the sense of being of service. To do "psycho-therapy" means that we pay attention to the psyche. When we give our attention to a person who is suffering or is in need of help it is not always a "set of techniques" that is most needed. Few would argue that therapeutic qualities of character such as emotional presence, emotional availability, maturity, commitment, courage, humour, awareness, etc., are best described as a set of techniques.

But what exactly is the *psyche* to which we give our attention and aim to serve? First of all it needs to be emphasised that the psyche is not identical to the mind. The Greek word *psyche* has three meanings. "Mind" is not one of them. If we want to be true to the essence of our calling we can state definitively that psychotherapy is not a branch of mental health. From this it follows that the psyche cannot be confined to the brain. Neuroscience explores the relationship of brain to mind but it leaves the greater part of the psyche untouched.

So again what is the "psyche"? Firstly it refers to the "soul". The soul is not the same as the brain or the mind. Neither can the soul be said to reside exclusively *in* the brain or the mind. We must also distinguish soul from "spirit" with which it is often confused. Western spiritual tradition imagines spirit in the heights. Heaven is above us. The Olympian gods of the Greeks lived on a mountain top. Angels have wings and bring their messages down to us from above. We imagine somehow that what is "high" is noble and desirable. The "highest" purpose of our "higher self" is the most worthy. We seek a "higher" perspective. What is "low" is of less worth and is perhaps best avoided.

We sometimes imagine that the psyche is located in or connected with the brain. The Greek word *menos* means both "spirit" and "mind". It is at the root of our words "mental" and "mind". It unites mind and spirit. In Homer's *Odyssey*, its hero Odysseus is at times guided by his wise and trusted friend Mentor. Mentor is a disguised form of Athene, a warrior goddess from high Olympus. Mentor can be seen as an early literary example of a wise spiritually aware counsellor. Practitioners who aim to bring clear thinking, higher perspective, and overview to guide those with troubled minds are perhaps the true "mental health practitioners". In the words of the Jungian scholar C. A. Meier "The brain is, for the most part, our psychic orientation system; it is by no means the psyche itself" (Meier, 1986, p. 268).

In myth Psyche thrives as a result of her encounter with the depths. A psychotherapy that is true to its etymological roots aims more to enable "under"—standing of issues than it aims to "over"—come them. Psyche was envisaged as a beautiful innocent young maid. She lived a charmed but ultimately unsatisfying life of blissful unconsciousness in which all her wishes were effortlessly fulfilled. Her growing discontent and curiosity required her to know more about her invisible lover with whom she lived in a magic castle. The jealous goddess Aphrodite determined she would gain awareness by a terrifying and apparently hopeless descent into the underworld. Only by this means and after her return to earth, could she find fulfilment in a conscious relationship to her lover.

Freud echoed the theme of descent. He envisaged psychotherapy as a downward journey into a frightening and disturbing underworld of chaotic primitive forces. In his view psyche required more than attendance and service. It needed the "liberation" that lies at the root of the word analysis (from the Greek "to unloose"). The patient journeyed downward to retrieve something of value lost amongst that which had been ignored, rejected, and forgotten. Freud's aim was to transform "hysterical misery into common unhappiness" (Freud, 1895d).

Psyche follows a different path to that of a masculine hero such as Odysseus who achieves his aim by strength and skill. She faces her trials without weapons and is unprepared for battle. She lacks the heroism of Odysseus who (aided by spiritual counselling) endures his trials with strength and ingenuity. He ultimately achieves a bloody victory over his enemies. Psyche faces the dark alone. She perseveres in the face of despair. Hers is the kind of courage we must all have in order to face those dark aspects of life and death over which we have little or no power. In the myth Psyche's courage and determination is rewarded by relational maturity rather than by a triumph of the will.

In keeping with the myth, psychotherapy welcomes and serves the psyche's need for descent and re-emergence. Our clients are likely to be those who are in some way low, feel "down", or overwhelmed. They may feel they have lost their standpoint or their standing in the world and want a new "under"-standing. We can assist them to "get to the bottom of things". Following the myth, we know that Psyche needs the dreaded downward journey to transform naivety and innocence into wisdom and the capacity to relate. We respect depth. We encourage and accompany those in need of this descent. We offer meaning and significance to this essential task. Yes, there is hope of return to the daylight.

There are of course many treatments, chemical and otherwise, that enable and even encourage us to avoid the dark descents that we associate with Psyche. We are told that fear, pain, loss, feelings of hopelessness, etc., can be avoided. Perhaps they can, at least for a time. However with our eye on the myth, we can see that these attempts are not "psychotherapeutic" in the root sense. If we try to enable Psyche to avoid her task, this will stunt her development and limit her capacity to mature. As professionals we may fear for Psyche and worry on her behalf. We may want to rescue her. This could perhaps be more for our own needs than for hers. We may offer her everything we can to keep her safely here with us. We may want to help her to keep on functioning in the everyday world just as she always used to. We may think it in her best interests to avoid going down. We may ourselves be under pressure from those who wish to avoid risk and demand predetermined results within predetermined times.

* * *

Psyche is also the Greek word for breath. Psyche (breath) is a state of perpetual exchange between the individual and the environment. That which is outside nourishes and sustains that which is within. That which is within nourishes and sustains that which is outside. The whole of the oxygen breathing animal kingdom is a part of evolution's answer to the danger of an over oxygenated atmosphere subject to combustion. We do our humble part to serve and protect the plant kingdom. Each breath maintains the symbiosis between the plant and animal kingdoms. In a sense each kingdom acts as the externalised organ of the other enabling the survival of both.

The psyche is the breath. Breath (psyche) is neither inside nor outside of us. Indeed it is not a thing at all. It is a process. There can be no psyche (breath) without the living body. Nor can there be breath (psyche) without an atmosphere to breathe. Psyche is simultaneously both inside and outside. It is not just contained within our skins or held within the brain. It is equally to be found in the world.

With this perpetual exchange in mind we cannot speak of psychological disorders as though they were to do with the individual alone. Terms such as post-traumatic stress disorder (PTSD), attention deficit hyperactivity disorder (ADHD), obsessive compulsive disorder (OCD), and seasonal affective disorder (SAD) isolate and alienate the individual. At the same time they inflate the importance of the individual. We make the client personally responsible for their failure to cope with the sometimes overpowering pathology of the environment. Those caught up in the overwhelming horrors of war for example might be considered to have a "disorder" (PTSD) on their return to a peaceful environment. Psychotherapeutic attention to the disordered social forces which create social conflict is largely absent. If we are mindful of the nature of psyche, we avoid creating such disconnections from the environment.

Psyche is breath. Every "disorder" has both an inner and an outer aspect. In addition to the attention we give the individual client we might also ask; what is it about the way our culture responds to and deals with trauma that leads to disorder? In what way is our culture disordered? Are our children overstimulated (perhaps by advertising and junk food) and insufficiently supported and contained? What is disordered in our society that allows this to be so? Why do we find it surprising that our bodies are affected by the seasons? Why do we regard it as a disorder to slow down and withdraw in the cold and dark of winter? What is our response to a culture that has lost its rituals and the traditions that recognise and contextualise the anxiety of normal human development? All of these terms imply that psychological attention needs to be directed toward the individual. Too often we first turn our gaze away from the psychic environment and then look to the disconnected individual for understanding.

By pathologising the individual rather than the environment we disconnect psyche from the world. Our definition of health can veer toward adjustment to social norms which may themselves be disordered. People who cannot tolerate the intolerable are not necessarily "disordered". Early breakdown of the individual in a dysfunctional system may well be a sign of health. If we lack the means to flee or to fight a damaging situation, breakdown may be the healthiest option. Paradoxically, the breakdown of the individual may be a sign of health for the system if it is willing and able to address its role in the breakdown. The individual "disorder" could lead to a healthier social order.

* * *

Psyche also has a third meaning. It is the word for butterfly. It seems that the psyche needs not only to breathe but also to fly. Psyche is identified with this delicate, fragile, attractive, fleeting, and colourful creature. The butterfly does not respond well to being pinned down. Scientific and logical attempts to grasp the psyche violate its essential nature in ways that endanger its existence.

With these etymological considerations in mind we can say that the *Diagnostic and Statistical Manual* (DSM) is not a friend of the living psyche. Yes, it may help to pin point and to identify particular symptoms and conditions but it does not address the psyche in any of the three root senses of the word. It addresses the mind rather than the psyche. It separates the individual from the environment. It pins its subject down in order to observe it closely thus denying the psyche its elusive character. We must follow rather than grasp the butterfly if we are to know it. We must appreciate that the psyche, in accord with its essential nature, takes us beyond what we can grasp or know. It must do. All our ways of thinking, feeling, sensing, imagining, and knowing are the stuff of which the psyche is made. Attempts to control or master the psyche will always fail. The part cannot grasp the whole.

Illness is a part of health

Health is a state of complete physical, mental, and social well-being and not merely the absence of disease or infirmity.

(World Health Organisation, 1946, p. 100)

The U.K. Health Professions Council was set up by a piece of legislation called the Health Professions Order in 2001. Until 2011 it was in negotiation with representatives of the psychotherapy profession over the way our occupation was best managed and regulated. One point of agreement did not seem to be contested. Along with paramedics, podiatrists, hearing aid dispensers, and twelve other health professions, psychotherapists were in agreement that they were indeed health care professionals. If this can be said to be the case it begs the question of what exactly do we all understand by the term "health".

As can be seen in the definition above, health professionals can have an idealised, even utopian, view of what constitutes health. This existing definition of health was formulated by the World Health Organisation back in 1948. It was an attempt to move away from a prevailing negative definition of health as being simply the absence of disease and infirmity. To be completely healthy, they decided, we must have a sense of well-being that extends beyond the physical, into the mental and on into the social/societal realms. Like all idealised and perfectionist aspirations the net effect of this is that it reminds the aspirant of his or her shortcomings and insufficiencies.

For this reason there is presently some debate amongst medical professionals as to whether the definition should be modified (Huber, 2011, p. 235). Many medics today are thinking that health might be better thought of as the ability to "adapt and self-manage" in order to retain our sense of "well-being". In other words those living with less than complete physical, psychological, and social well-being might still consider themselves to be healthy so long as they can self-manage and find a sense of adequate well-being despite their imperfections. Patients or clients might in turn settle for the much more achievable end of having a state of health that Donald Winnicott might have called "good enough". Obviously this possible new definition would take considerable stress off health care providers allowing them to be less heroic.

As health professionals we may continue to consider illness to be the enemy as we do in the present definition of health. Alternatively we might learn to live relatively contentedly with a certain degree of less than ideal health while enjoying a satisfactory sense of well-being. Illness according to both of these views remains something to be over-come and ideally avoided. This apparently attractive objective is spoiled only by the fact that it is impossible. Not one of us will leave this life in a "state of complete physical, mental, and social well-being and not merely the absence of disease or infirmity". Death and disease are a part of living a whole life.

So what is "health"? Etymologically health means "wholeness". To "heal" is to "make whole or healthy". As healing professionals we must learn to accept illness (and indeed death) in the interests of wholeness. Health accordingly cannot be an "absence of illness or infirmity". On the contrary health must allow for the presence of illness and infirmity.

Well-being is not the same as health

Curiously the World Health Organisation defines health (wholeness) in terms of "well-being". Whatever can be meant by well-being? The English word "well" can be traced back to its Latin root "velle" which means "to wish strongly". It is related to the word "volition" which means "the act of exercising the will". In effect the medical definition of health refers to a state in which we feel as we want to feel or would wish to feel.

Those psychotherapists and others with an awareness of unconscious and subliminal psychological processes will immediately have a problem with this. What part of the psyche is doing the wishing and the wanting? We are aware that the psyche is made of many parts. Many therapies hypothesise that the psyche is made of conscious, semi-conscious, and unconscious aspects. According to theory these can have very different wishes and desires. Are we saying then that health is a kind of ego gratification? What gratifies one part of the psyche may create problems for another part. What if we want both security and freedom for instance? What if a client enjoys the longed for success of a career breakthrough and suddenly becomes inexplicably depressed upon achieving this. The depth psychological work might be to explore the losses of freedom that accompany the new responsibilities and the emotional repercussions of this.

Some therapies address symptoms but do not recognise the significance of unconscious processes. In cases of depression for example therapies and medical prescriptions for antidepressants might lead to a greater sense well-being. The patient or client may feel more as he or she wishes to feel or believes he or she should feel but it does not lead to greater wholeness. The depression might in fact be a positive and purposive sign that something is missing from consciousness that needs to be included in order to gain "wholeness" (or health). If conscious awareness is not complete or whole it cannot be described as "healthy". The feeling of improved well-being gained by such medical or psychological interventions may further the wishes of the conscious ego but can only be described as "un-healthy" in as far as it blocks the unconscious concerns that would "heal" the psyche and make it more whole.

Holism

Apart from the fact that there is no mention of soul or spirit, the World Health Organisation's definition of health cannot be faulted with regard to its holism and ambition. Physical, psychological, and social aspects are given equal status. It follows from this that the Health Professions Council is justified in bringing together counsellors and psychotherapists who deal mainly with the psychological facets of health with paramedics, podiatrists, hearing aid dispensers, and others who are in the main concerned with the more physical aspects. In accord with this line of thinking the HPC may at some point wish to consider achieving an even more holistic approach. It could also be monitoring and regulating professions that deal with the social dimensions of health. Amongst others, these professions might include social workers, teachers, police, and politicians. It is interesting to consider how politicians might respond to being monitored by regulators who include psychotherapists.

When we consider health from this holistic perspective of the physical, psychological, and social we can see that what happens to us in one of these three domains may have its roots in another. The patient who presents to the doctor with a physical illness such as diabetes may perhaps trace its origins to a weight problem. This in turn may have emotional, familial, social, or political roots. Perhaps a habit of comfort eating developed as a strategy for dealing with unmet emotional needs. These in turn might be the by-product of social and financial disadvantages suffered by the parents of the patient, or of social pressures that result in poor diet.

In our fragmented health care system and with a fragmented view of health there is likelihood that a medical practitioner will be unaware of the emotional underpinnings of a physical disease. A physician may not be able to imagine more deeply into a condition like diabetes other than considering its biochemical and dietary implications. Psychotherapists may be equally unaware of the implications of medical treatments.

Physicians and psychotherapists share alike the experience of most often working one-on-one with their patients or clients. Both are unlikely to know their patient or client in a social context. It is difficult for them to see illness and symptoms in their wider context. Marital, family, group, and systemic therapists will have a broader outlook but none will come near to addressing health as "complete social well-being".

Health is paradoxical

Given that illness and death cannot be eliminated or avoided we must accept them as inescapable realities of life. We could consider that there are healthy and unhealthy responses to these realities. Examples of unhealthy responses might include denial, nihilism, or despair. Passive and resigned acceptance of ill health could also be considered as another way of refusing to engage with the energies of illness. So also could be clinging to the symptoms and sufferings of illness in order to gain practical or psychological advantages. All of these responses amount to unawareness, inability, or refusal to see meaning and significance in the challenges that illness presents. We cannot see the bigger picture and so respond in an unhealthy way. That is to say in a way that does not consider the whole of the situation.

A more holistic approach and in terms of this discussion a more "healthy" approach might involve receptivity, acceptance, interest, and a willingness to engage in a dynamic interaction with the energy behind illness. We would do this knowing that the illness may contain the potential to make us more whole. This brings us to another nuance in our exploration of the words "health" and "wholeness". We now meet the missing spiritual and soul element in the World Health Organisation's definition. "Wholeness" is closely related to "holiness". The Western medical tradition has spiritual roots. It is descended from the times of Hippocrates and the ancient Greek healing temples sacred to the god Asklepios. Healing was then regarded as a spiritual act facilitated by doctors who were also priests. Our nursing profession retains something of this tradition with its ecclesiastical history. The eleventh century Sufi mystic and intellectual Abu Hamid al-Ghazali said "Illness is one of the forms of experience by which humans arrive at a knowledge of God; as He says, 'Illnesses are my servants which I attach to my chosen friends'" (1909, p. 42). In the modern era C. G. Jung made a similar remark when he said that in today's world the gods have become diseases.

The notion that afflictions are a divine privilege is not an easy one for patient, client, doctor, or psychotherapist. Yet it is widely recognised. In the Sri Lankan healing tradition for example the spirits of illness are recognised as being ultimately in the service of the Buddha; while in the Christian tradition we can relate to the frustration of St Theresa of Avila. This devout sixteenth century Carmelite nun was afflicted by bouts of malaria. Once when travelling, her cart broke and tipped her into a muddy stream. She is reputed to have cried out to God "If this is the way you treat your friends it is no wonder you have so few of them!"

Illness can be seen as a way of putting us in touch with disassociated and/or emerging aspects of our being. These may originate primarily in the body, the mind, the social being, or in matters of spirit. A "healthy" response would be to bring the new experience into association with other aspects of our being. Illness is physical but not just physical, psychological but not just psychological, social but not just social, and spiritual but not just spiritual. To make and to see these connections is to step toward a more holistic view. To facilitate such connecting is an act of "making whole" or healing. It is a step toward health.

Illness is a part of the human experience. Life is ever evolving. Balances shift. Dis-ease is an inevitable part of this process. Constant adaptations are necessary in order to function successfully and to live fully in a fluctuating world. Illness stops us in our tracks, disrupts habitual behaviours, and forces new behaviours and adaptations. It can also expand our capacity to feel and invite us to adopt new ways of thinking. Health is more than a sense of well-being. Health is less about feeling good and more about being whole and responsible (able to respond) to life. To do this we must not only accept the inevitability of illness but learn to value it as a part of health.

CHAPTER TWO

Imaginal healing

Carl Jung stressed the idea that "Image is psyche", (1931a, p. 130). He insisted that, "Every psychic process is an image and an imagining" (1958, p. 544). However, the English language can make it difficult for us to discuss the power and potency of the imagination. We are limited by the long held cultural presupposition that something which is "imaginary" is also something that is "unreal". Furthermore we are inclined to suppose that the imagination is a subordinate aspect of the psyche in mature healthy adults. It is something that we "have". We forget and overlook the fact that the imagination might be better understood as something that "has us". For sure, the dispassionate objective scientist imagines the world in very different ways to that of an impassioned religious fundamentalist; but both see the world through the power of the imagination. The results that they produce for good or for ill will be a consequence of their style of imagination. These different "styles" of imagining the world about us and which have us in their thrall (very often unconsciously) used to be called the "gods".

For this reason the French philosopher and theologian Henry Corbin found it necessary to invent a word that would not trivialise the "imaginary" as something insubstantial and subservient to the ego. He coined the word "imaginal" as an alternative, in order to describe this deeper understanding of the imagination as a potent force that enables us to perceive and to respond to our world.

Bearing these considerations in mind we can look at the phenomenon of the placebo and remain open to the possibility that placebos can offer far more than just an insubstantial, illusory, or "imaginary" benefit to our health.

The Powerful Placebo

One should treat as many patients as soon as possible with the new drug while it still has the power to heal. (2008, p. 126)

Sir William Osler (known as the father
of Western medicine)

In April 1960 the *American Journal of Cardiology* published the results of a test on an innovative new surgical technique designed to help sufferers of pain from angina pectoris (Kaptchuk, 1986, pp. 102–105). This is a condition in which a sufferer is subject to sudden intense chest pains caused by a momentary lack of adequate blood supply to the heart. The technique was called "mammary artery ligation". This procedure involved shutting off a perfectly good artery in order to encourage the body to use smaller arteries to feed the heart. The technique had been used for some years. Both patients and doctors reported an eighty percent success rate. This was judged by the subjective feelings of the patients and by objective clinical measurement.

Researchers at the University of Kansas Medical Center decided to check the validity of these impressive results in a different way. To do this they used a method that would not be acceptable according to present day medical ethics. They set up what is called a "double blind" test. Patients were admitted and prepared in every way for surgery. At the operating table a card was drawn which determined by a fifty/fifty chance whether or not the patient would actually be given the procedure. Patients who were not given the procedure were instead marked with a scalpel to create a scar that would be indistinguishable from that of the patients who had actually been given the operation. None of the hospital staff knew which patients were which. All of those in the operating theatre had been sworn to secrecy and were not permitted to interact with the patients after the operation.

All of the patients, regardless of whether or not they had had the operation, demonstrated a forty percent improvement by objective clinical tests and measurements. Those who had had the operation reported a seventy-six percent improvement in their sense of wellbeing. However, those who had merely had the scar and no operation at all reported a one hundred percent improvement.

Despite the clear evidence based success both by objective and subjective measures the procedure came to be regarded as a failure. Surgery had been shown to be no more effective than a mere scar. The technique was therefore abandoned. The patients it seemed had healed in the wrong way and for the wrong reasons. This could not be condoned by the scientifically based medical profession. The patients had improved due to the placebo effect.

* * *

A more recent study published in 2002 has thrown doubt on the need for certain expensive medical procedures. A common procedure known as partial meniscectomy is used to treat people suffering with knee problems. It involves treating tears in the cartilage between the upper and lower portions of the knee joints. This is done either by a technique called lavage, which involves flushing out bad cartilage with liquid, or by debridement which entails cutting away loose or worn cartilage which is thought to cause pain and restrict mobility. The procedures are evidently effective and are offered to up to 700,000 people a year in the USA alone at an annual cost of some four billion dollars.

However in 2002 research was conducted which divided 180 osteoarthritis patients randomly into three groups of equal numbers. It tested the effectiveness of the two techniques against a placebo group who were merely scarred with a scalpel. A two year follow-up study showed that patients in all three groups reported an equal degree of improvement in pain reduction and mobility (Mosely, 2002, pp. 81–82). These results have been further backed up by a Finnish study published in 2013 (Sihvonen et al., 2013).

Another study found that heart patients who had received pacemaker implantation achieved benefits that were demonstrable by both objective and subjective measures whether or not their pacemakers had actually been switched on (Linde, 1999, pp. 903–907).

Pharmaceuticals

In 2003 a senior executive of GlaxoSmithKline, Dr. Allen Roses declared publicly that, "The vast majority of drugs—more than ninety per cent—only work for thirty or fifty per cent of people" (McGreevy, 2003). GlaxoSmithKline is Britain's largest pharmaceutical company. At the time he made this statement it had an annual turnover of thirty-one point eight billion pounds. If he is correct, it would seem that we might be entitled to suppose that over half this sum has been spent on ineffective medications.

Furthermore there has been some strong and extensive criticism of the way that research findings for drug trials are presented to the medical profession. The medic and writer Ben Goldacre says that:

> Drugs are tested by the people who manufacture them, in poorly designed trials, on hopelessly small numbers of weird, unrepresentative patients, and analysed using techniques which are flawed by design, in such a way that they exaggerate the benefits of treatments. Unsurprisingly these results favour the manufacturer. When trials throw up results that companies don't like, they are perfectly entitled to hide them from doctors and patients, so we only ever see a distorted picture of any drug's true effects. (2012, p. X)

He goes on to question the objectivity of some academic papers pointing out that they are on occasions "covertly planned and written by people who work for drug companies". Some academic journals, he says, are owned by a single drug company. It is clear that the perceived potency and effectiveness of some medications is exaggerated by these worrying distortions.

In the USA around ten per cent of the population over the age of six (yes, six) take antidepressant medication (Robson-Scott, 2011). In the UK doctors write some twenty-three million prescriptions for antidepressants each year. Research conducted by Irving Kirsch, a psychologist at the University of Connecticut concludes that:

> [...] compared with placebo, the new generation of antidepressants do not produce clinically significant improvements in depression in patients who initially have moderate or even severe depression, but show significant effects only in the most severely depressed

patients. The findings also show that the effects for these patients seem to be due to decreased responsiveness to placebo rather than increased responsiveness to medication. (Kirsch et al., 2008, pp. 11–21)

Similarly the British National Institute for Health and Clinical Excellence (NICE) is unable to prove that selective serotonin reuptake inhibitors (SSRIs) are better than placebo in achieving remission of depression (Agius, 2008, p. 22).

Bearing in mind the enormous costs incurred by medical treatments that in some cases show little or no better results than placebo treatments we might also want to consider research which indicates that placebos perform better the more they cost. Research at Massachusetts Institute of Technology in the USA found that eighty-five per cent of people given a "pain killer" placebo that they believed was priced at two dollars and fifty cents a tablet experienced a reduction in pain. Of a group who were given the same placebo remedy but who believed they were receiving a pain killing tablet that had been reduced in price to only ten cents a tablet only sixty-one per cent experienced pain reduction (Bates, 2008).

In recognition of the power and effectiveness of placebo medication a recent report commission by the German Medical Association (BÄK) revealed that half of all general practitioners in Germany have prescribed placebo drugs to their patients (Hughs, 2011). In Bavaria the figure is even higher at eighty-eight per cent.

We could of course question the ethics of deceiving a patient with a dummy medication, albeit a harmless one that as we have seen above, can be shown to be demonstrably and measurably effective. On the other hand we could also question professionals who are aware of the demonstrable potency of the placebo effect and yet continue to prescribe and administer expensive treatments that are known to be scarcely, if any, more potent than placebo and carry with them harmful side effects.

It is generally assumed to be the case that the potency of the placebo effect depends on the patient's belief that he or she is receiving a scientifically bona fide surgery or drug and not merely a superficial cut to the skin or a sugar pill. However there is research that indicates that this is not necessarily the case. Research at the Harvard Medical School's Osher Research Center shows evidence to the contrary. Eighty patients with irritable bowel syndrome (IBS) were divided into two equal groups. One group was not treated at all while the other received placebo pills. Professor Ted Kaptchuk who led the experiment explains that

> Not only did we make it absolutely clear that the pills had no active ingredient and were made from inert substances, but we actually had "placebo" printed on the bottle. We told the patients that they didn't have to even believe in the placebo effect. Just take the pills. (Cameron, 2010)

Over a three week period twice as many patients who had used the placebo reported adequate symptom relief than did those who had not been treated. What is more, Kaptchuk says that according to:

> [...] other outcome measures, patients taking the placebo doubled their rates of improvement to a degree roughly equivalent to the effect of the most powerful IBS medication. (Cameron, 2010)

It seems that any treatment which does not actually cause harm is better than no treatment at all. This point was brought home to me when working with David, a GP client in psychotherapy. All GPs including David are of course aware that the prescription of antibiotics is ineffective in treating a viral infection such as the common cold. Yet David confessed that he would do exactly this. He would prescribe himself a course of antibiotics because, despite the science of which he was perfectly aware, it "seemed to make him feel better".

What is more, when we consider the effectiveness of any treatment, medical or placebos, we must be mindful that the body can in time heal itself with no external treatment at all. Many patients visit their physician when their illness is at its climax. At this point improvement can often be expected without the aid of medications of any kind.

Psychotherapy

We have seen that a surgical procedure can have a discernibly positive outcome both objectively and subjectively, yet still be demonstrated to be a placebo. Studies show that antidepressant medication can have a seventy per cent positive outcome. Yet this too cannot be demonstrated to be significantly more effective than placebo (Robin-Scott, 2011).

How then can we possibly assess whether psychotherapy offers anything more than placebo? Unlike a surgical technique we cannot arrange for two identical sessions to be set up; one with a real trained experienced psychotherapist using real interventions and one with an unqualified inexperienced actor doing all the same things but merely pretending to be a psychotherapist. Nor is it possible to measure such stated therapeutic aims as individuation, self-actualisation or personal growth. Much less can we comment on the state of the soul; for "soul" is after all a root meaning of the word *psyche*. Soul cannot be quantified and measured. Yet government bodies in Britain confidently say that they base their support and funding for psychological intervention on "evidence based practice".

They are of course referring to much simpler, reductionist, and more easily measured outcomes. These include the lessening of presenting symptoms and a client's greater sense of wellbeing as a result of treatment. Are there fewer anxiety attacks? Has the depression been lifted? If so by how much can this be demonstrated on a scale of one to ten? Can the same result be achieved more quickly and cheaply by a drug prescription?

We have noted that medicine does not recognise a difference between wellbeing and health. A healthy response to a crisis or other difficulty in life is not necessarily a feeling of wellbeing or pleasurable contentment. We can recall Aldous Huxley's novel *Brave New World* in which the citizenry are kept in a permanent state of wellbeing with the aid of a drug called *soma*. Only the unhappy socially alienated hero could be described as "healthy". The novel makes it abundantly clear that wellbeing is not synonymous with "health". Medics are unlikely to share Freud's therapeutic objective of changing neurotic misery into "ordinary unhappiness". Nor are they likely to recognise the possibility of what psychoanalysts call a "flight into health". This concept proposes that in some circumstances patients may obtain sudden and otherwise inexplicable relief from symptoms when they are on the cusp of facing painful but potentially healing issues that may underlie their symptoms. A patient may suddenly find it more tolerable or even agreeable to dwell in depression or an anxiety state than to have to deal with the complexities that may follow from becoming conscious of the fact that their relationship or job can no longer meet their emotional needs. This provides a rationale to end the therapy before the painful issues are faced and dealt with. Sometimes it seems that we prefer the neurotic misery to the ordinary unhappiness. If we are successful in reducing symptoms by avoidance or suppression we may score well on the evidence base. Clients, patients, and funders may be pleased but we will not have "attended to the soul", raised awareness, or taken a step toward greater health or wholeness. An opportunity to do so will have been lost. What the medic may regard as a victory may be the psychotherapist's defeat and vice versa.

There are numerous studies that measure symptom relief and feelings of wellbeing (Eyesenck, 1952, pp. 319–324; Seligman, 1995, pp. 965–974; Smith, 1977, pp. 752–760). These consistently show that all schools of psychotherapy perform about as well as one another. Furthermore according to these criteria they perform little better than does medication or regular visits to the family doctor, a social worker, or according to one study—a university professor (Strupp, 1979, pp. 1125–1136). There is little evidence, according to these measures, to suggest that training in psychotherapy, years of personal therapy on the part of the practitioner, or supervision of psychotherapy practice are of consequence to the treatment outcome. There is no evidence to support the notion that cognitive behavioural therapy outperforms other approaches. If CBT has an advantage it would seem to be that it is particularly comfortable validating its results in terms of symptom removal and improved feelings of wellbeing. It doesn't achieve these goals any more effectively than other approaches do. If we agree that health is the same as wellbeing then psychotherapy can congratulate itself that in general it performs no worse and possibly, depending on the research criteria, even a little bit better than alternative treatments on offer.

It is unsurprising that government bodies and insurance companies are eager to save money by getting people back to work and normal functioning. Indeed a great many clients come to psychotherapy with these goals in mind. However, social norms can be and often are themselves dysfunctional. Norms can be unhealthy or "disordered" (to use the word favoured by those who aspire toward normalising). Normal functioning is not the main aim of a psychotherapy that works with the concept of the unconscious. In psychotherapy the symptom can be regarded as an indicator of deeper unconscious issues that need to come more fully into consciousness in order to promote wholeness or health. Many psychotherapists would no more wish to remove a symptom before addressing its underlying issue than a mechanic would wish to extinguish the warning light on an automobile dashboard without investigating the cause of the warning. In Georg Groddeck's words psychotherapy's aim is "to correctly interpret that which […] is trying to express (itself) through symptoms and to teach it a less painful mode of self-expression" (Ramos, 2004, p. 40).

This lessening of pain will of course create an enhanced feeling of wellbeing. This is rightly valued by doctors, healthcare funders, and patients alike. All of these are likely to desire a return to a familiar normality. We have seen that psychotherapists can be shown to do this as well as anyone. However, for psychotherapists who hold a depth perspective the aim is greater than this. Deep changes will almost certainly involve upsetting the status quo. Problems and emotions that have been avoided may need to be confronted and dealt with. Life may never be the same again when a patient confronts that which is deeply within. Unlike the physician or the social worker the aim of the psychotherapist is to bring the limited ego into contact with those unknown forces which impinge upon it in the form of symptoms. The aim is to find a way of living with more integrity and authenticity whilst admitting reality more fully. Reality, authenticity, and integrity are not qualities that lend themselves to the kind of measurement demanded by a government agency or an insurance company's evidence base.

Nocebos

To the extent that we can deal with the placebo element in both medicine and psychotherapy we must address a further complication. Placebo (Latin for "I will please") has a shadow side which is less well known. Put in dramatic terms we might even call it an "evil twin". This is the nocebo (Latin for "I will harm"). In this case it is an effect that occurs when a patient is given a medication or told something that should make no difference whatsoever to their health; but ends up causing negative side effects due to what they believe about the medicine they are taking or what is said to them.

For obvious reasons this effect is much more difficult to demonstrate. Bound by Hippocrates' injunction to "first do no harm" health professionals are not in a position to easily explore the nocebo. However this is not to say that it had not been done. For instance an Italian study found that twenty-seven per cent of participants with drug allergies would develop the same side effects if given a dummy pill instead of the medication to which they were allergic (Liccardi et al., 2004, pp. 104–107).

Another trial found that patients reported the same side effects whether they received an anticonvulsant medication or a placebo (Amanzio et al., 2009, pp. 261–269).

If an expectation of negative consequences can lead to those results becoming manifest how far can this principle be applied? In 1992 the *Southern Medical Journal* reported the case of a man who had been diagnosed with metastatic carcinoma of the oesophagus. He, his family, and his physician all believed he was dying of widespread cancer. He duly died as expected. At his autopsy only a two centimetre nodule of cancer in his liver was found. His intern, Clifton Meador, did not believe he died of cancer. "Could it be his expectation of death that killed him?" he wondered (Meador, 1992, p. 246). If such negative side effects and even death are a factor contributing to these results then clearly nocebo is an issue that we must take seriously. To this end many doctors avoid drawing attention to painful and uncomfortable side effects that can accompany surgeries and medications. Research has shown that these effects are likely to increase if a patient's attention is drawn to them.

Another dramatic example of probable nocebo effect occurred amongst Laotian refugees who were resettled in the United States after the Vietnam War. Members of the Hmong ethnic group had fought a guerrilla war against the government of Laos with US backing. When the Laotian communist government won the war many Hmong took refuge in the USA to avoid reprisals. The American government decided to scatter the refugees randomly across the country to fifty-three different cities; thus breaking up the cultural integrity of the group. This further compounded the problems of a people who had a strong sense of tradition. In their own country they lived close to the land as farmers and hunters and had deeply held animistic as well as Christian beliefs.

Within a matter of months of arrival in their new country there were a large number of unexplained deaths that occurred amongst the migrants while they slept. The phenomenon occurred regardless of where they had been resettled. All but one of the 117 deaths were among healthy men with a median age of thirty-three years. The medical profession could offer no explanation. They could only respond by labelling the phenomenon as Sudden Unexplained Nocturnal Death Syndrome or SUNDS.

One migrant was able to offer an explanation. He said that:

> When the Hmong don't worship properly, do not perform religious
> ritual properly or forget to sacrifice or whatever, then the ancestor
> spirits or the village spirits do not want to guard them. That's why
> the evil spirit is able to come and get them. (Madrigal, 2011)

At that time and place it was the case that for a great number of reasons the Hmong were not able to abide by their traditions and perform the rituals that they believed were essential to their survival and wellbeing. To all appearances it seemed that the uniting thread that joined the SUNDS victims was the cultural belief system that they shared in common. It seems that they were mortally endangered by the cultural belief system which held the view that they were in mortal danger.

In psychotherapy as in medicine we must be aware of the dangerous nocebo potential of diagnosis. Psychiatrist Eileen Walkenstein summed the matter up admirably well in the title of her book *Shrunk to Fit.* Psychiatric labelling diminishes and confines the person who is labelled. It can evoke and foster the very conditions it claims to address. A condition is not the same as a personal identity. It follows that there is in fact no such thing as a schizophrenic, a depressive, a masochist, a hysteric, an anorexic, a bulimic, and so on. Says Walkenstein:

> A psychiatric diagnosis is like a jail sentence, a permanent mark
> on your record that follows wherever you go. And even though
> psychiatrists know how little value there is in their diagnosis, they
> persist in playing Judge, handing down sentences.
>
> In my psychiatric residency we were taught "once a
> schizophrenic, always a schizophrenic." This, a life sentence, a sentence for life, attacking and replacing a life, despite the common
> experience that you couldn't get two psychiatrists to agree on any
> one diagnosis at one time. (1975, p. 22)

She goes on to comment that she had often heard her professional colleagues say with "a mixture of disgust, contempt and repulsion [...] 'Ahh, he's just a schizophrenic.'" Clearly what she is describing here is not a dispassionate scientific medical diagnosis. It has something of the character of what used to be called a curse. In the context of this discussion we shall call it a nocebo. The opprobrium that attends the diagnostic label is only likely to compound the patient's difficulties.

The sometimes arbitrary but adhesive nature of psychiatric diagnosis was explored by psychologist David Rosenhan. In 1973 he performed a couple of experiments to illustrate this point (1973, pp. 250–258). He and a number of his colleagues claimed to be experiencing auditory hallucinations in order to gain admission into a number of mental hospitals. All were diagnosed and admitted. Once in, they behaved perfectly normally and said that their hallucinations had stopped. Their normal behaviours however continued to be interpreted by staff as symptoms of mental illness. As a condition of their release all were forced to admit that they were mentally ill and to agree to take antipsychotic drugs.

One of the offended hospitals challenged Rosenhan to send pseudo patients to them. They were convinced that they would be easily identified. He agreed to do this. In the following weeks out of 195 new admissions, the hospital staff identified forty-one people as pseudo patients. Rosenhan had sent no one to the hospital.

In psychotherapy both the therapist and the client can anticipate, magnify, and selectively attend to the issues that a diagnosis suggests. If the diagnosis suggests a poor outcome, this can become an additional impediment to the client. It is even more likely to become a self-fulfilling prophesy if family, friends, and employers share the bad news. Expectations have consequences for both good and ill. Placebo and nocebo responses are not insubstantial delusions afforded to gullible and malleable people. Indeed there is some evidence that indicates that the body can learn how to heal itself under the guidance, as it were, of a placebo. In the 1970s experiments were done to measure the effect of an anticancer drug called cyclophosphamine. This drug has the effect of suppressing the immune system. The drug was repeatedly given to mice in combination with saccharine. The effects were measured and the immune systems of the mice were observed. The findings indicated that the drug had the desired effect of lowering immunity. Eventually the researchers stopped administering the drug and gave the mice saccharine alone. It was discovered that the mice continued to respond as though they had received the drug. It appeared that the cells had learned to perform the work of the drug unaided by the drug itself. They needed only the cue of the placebo/nocebo in order to produce the required effect (Sternberg, 2001, pp. 159–181).

It is clear that the placebo effect has genuine measurable objective and subjective results. Placebos have far more consequence than is normally attributed to them. In part due to ethical restraints many of our major medical procedures have not undergone double-blind studies. In many cases the placebo effect can be as high as seventy per cent. It is therefore unknown to what extent any scientifically validated evidence based practice that has not been validated by a double-blind study is justified. Perhaps such an untested evidence base is in itself a foundation for a placebo effect. Maybe it is our very confidence and irrational belief in scientific medicine that gives it much of its potency.

We can see from the collected evidence that many patients benefit from placebos. It is not so much the case that they imagine that their condition has improved as it is that their condition has improved due to the power of their imagination.

CHAPTER THREE

Signs, symptoms, and metaphors

Sigmund Freud believed that pathology was the key to understanding the unconscious psyche. He went so far as to declare that, "We can catch the unconscious only in pathological material" (1965, p. 64).

When we use the word "symptom" we refer to "any sensation or change in bodily function that is associated with a particular disease" or to "any phenomenon or circumstance accompanying something and regarded as evidence of its existence" (Makins, 1979, p. 1652). The word derives from the Greek "sumptōma" meaning "a coincidence" or "to fall together" (Partridge, 1958, p. 689).

Patients tend to consult physicians and psychotherapists when they suffer physical or psychological symptoms. It is our symptoms that prompt us to look for help from a health consultant. Symptoms are dynamic and motivational. They impose themselves upon our consciousness. They create worry. They demand attention. Things are not as we feel they should be. Maybe we suffer dizziness, anxiety, depression, sleeplessness, headaches, heart palpitations, stomach complaints, eczema, etc. What does the symptom indicate? What is it in the body or the psyche that needs attention? Is there a cream or a salve, a pill, or a therapy that will put an end to the distress?

Medicine is however less interested in our symptoms than it is in actual "signs" of illness and disease. It is possible for a patient to suffer unpleasant and disabling symptoms such as those above and yet to have no identifiable illness. On the other hand it is perfectly possible for a patient to be free of symptoms, to enjoy a sense of wellbeing, and yet be detected to have a disease or illness such as hypertension. Medicine distinguishes the identifiable "signs" that point to illnesses from symptoms that have no detectable physical cause. Identifiable illnesses can be treated. Symptoms are subjective. From the point of view of biological medicine they are "mere" subjective symptoms unless and until they can be validated as signs.

From a medical point of view, these lesser purely symptomatic ailments might be suitable for treatment by alternative health practitioners. Practitioners such as faith healers, homeopaths, past life regression therapists, psychotherapists, and counsellors, etc., who work outside of the rigorous hard evidence based discipline of scientific medicine might yet be able to provide some help to distressed patients who have no identifiable physical illness. This is all the better of course, if they can provide an "evidence base" to demonstrate the effectiveness of their treatment in relieving or eliminating symptoms. This evidence will need to compare favourably with psychotropic medications with regard to cost effectiveness and timescale.

Halfway through the twentieth century psychopharmacology began to designate a kind of intermediate class of symptoms. These were treated as "signs" of conditions that might otherwise be regarded as purely symptomatic. It was discovered for instance that manic depressive illness or bipolar mood swings would respond to treatment by lithium carbonate. In minimal amounts lithium is a naturally occurring element in the body. It is not however believed to perform any biological function (Jeanty, 2014). The large, dangerous, near toxic doses which are necessary to stabilise mood swings require careful monitoring to prevent damage to the liver. The cause of bipolar disorder remains unknown. It is not able to be detected other than by its symptoms of mood swings. It is not in any way caused by a lithium deficiency.

Similarly today, despite the widespread use of selective serotonin reuptake inhibitor (SSRI) antidepressants and anxiety medications, there is no evidence that depression and anxiety are caused by a deficiency in serotonin levels (Dach, 2014). All that is known is that an abundance of serotonin promotes a feeling of wellbeing. SSRI medications such as Prozac, Zoloft, and Paxil, etc., have been shown in trials to be scarcely more effective than a placebo (Kirsch et al., 2008, pp. 11–21) and are known to come at the expense of side effects such as nausea, constipation, and sexual impotence. The causes of depression and anxiety remain unknown by medical science. Depression cannot be demonstrated by a blood test. It remains a purely symptomatic illness.

Symptoms and symbols

If psychotherapy's main task is to "attend to the psyche" as the word itself suggests, it will be somewhat out of step with medical priorities. We will not necessarily equate symptom removal with health. We will be interested in what unconscious material lies behind the symptom. Unlike medics we will not feel that it is our role to regard the symptom as a possible "sign". That is the sphere of medicine. We will instead look to the symptom as a possible "symbol" (Greek; *sumbolon* "to throw, hence put together, to compare"). We will be interested in the symptom not as a mere coincidence but regard it symbolically, as meaningfully connected to an underlying condition.

Like Freud we will aim to "catch the unconscious [...] in pathological material". We will concur with James Hillman that "the psyche dos not exist without pathologising" (1975, p. 70). Like Georg Groddeck we will see our primary role as being "to correctly interpret that which [...] is trying to express (itself) through symptoms and to teach it a less painful mode of self-expression" (Ramos, 2004, p. 40). Psychotherapy has a fundamentally different role to that of medicine, a different perspective, and different priorities. Psychotherapy is not a junior profession to medicine. It has its own purpose, tasks, and responsibilities. It has its own definition of health; a definition that allows for wholeness and makes room for the inevitable and unavoidable sufferings and strife of a fully lived life. Unlike the medical profession we do not long for or aim toward the perfectionist ideal of "complete physical, mental, and social wellbeing and not merely the absence of disease or infirmity" (World Health Organisation, 1946, p. 100).

It is regrettable that the psychotherapy profession seems in many instances to have willingly surrendered its capacity to challenge or explore its relationship with the predominant medical, economic, and academic model of health. Instead we find ourselves struggling to demonstrate convincingly that we are effective at removing symptoms quickly and cost effectively. Too often we seem to prefer to do this than to contest this shallow and incomplete model of health. In return, at least up to now, the profession has enjoyed the benefits of secure paid work from health care providers, academic institutions, and insurance companies. If we share medicine's ambitious aim of eliminating symptoms and pathological material then according to Freud and Hillman we also lose our connection to the unconscious psyche. We then cease to be psychotherapists in any meaningful sense of the word. We can join Jung in his lament from the 1930's that we are acceding to a "psychology without the psyche" (1931b, p. 344).

Symptoms as opportunity

How then does psychotherapy go about its task of finding meaning in a symptom? First of all in psychotherapy the symptom is not seen as the enemy. Our first aim is not to suppress or eliminate the symptom. Instead we can value it as we might value a dream. We can hear it as a voice of unconscious processes which are announcing their presence to the consciousness of the client. Paradoxically the psychotherapist can provide some immediate relief to the client in this way by taking on board some the function of the symptom. We ourselves can begin to act as a bridge between the conscious and unconscious processes with which we are presented. The client speaks to us with two voices; the voice of the conscious known "problem" or issue and the voice of the symptom which speaks on behalf of the unconscious. We listen to both presentations with equal interest and attentiveness.

Jung defines the psyche as "the totality of all psychic processes, conscious as well as unconscious" (1921, p. 463). The psychotherapist then sees the symptom as not "just" a symptom (i.e., a "coincidence"). It becomes a meaningful symbol (i.e., something that is "put" together). In the case of depression we are interested in and sympathetic to what is being depressed or "pressed down" by the conscious ego. How can we allow it to come up and make its voice heard? In the case of panic attacks we are interested to know why the client is being attacked by his or her own nature. Pan is the old Greek god of nature and woodlands. Why is he intruding into consciousness and scuppering normal life?

The symptom is not the same as the problem. Sometimes a disabling symptom or ill health is the best solution to a problem that the psyche has so far been able to devise. How else does one deal with an impossible situation? Perhaps we have a persecutory manager at work. Confrontation or complaint may lead to unemployment. Jobs may be scarce. Our financial responsibilities may be great. In this case the true pathology that needs to be addressed may be a social one. A workforce of employees who function with symptoms suppressed whilst being propped up by medications may simply allow an intolerable situation to persist. Such a toxic work environment may create a necessity for even more serious and insistent illnesses to bring it to an end. We might go so far as to agree with Abraham Maslow when he says that:

> [...] the concepts of sickness and health may fuse and blur when we see the symptom as a pressure toward health, or see the neurosis as the healthiest possible solution at the moment to the problem of the individual. (1968, p. 92)

How does one deal with one's own "inner voices" that lead to unrealistic self-expectations? These may perhaps derive from over demanding emotionally unavailable parent figures. In this case the client's issues are essentially the parents' issues; parents who may have long since died. A client may have to rethink and redeem the parents' values in order to be freed of these inner voices and discover her or his own. In such a case Pan may be calling a client back to their own truer and deeper nature. Medication may block this process. Depression and anxiety can have the beneficial effect of removing us from such an impossible situation by creating opportunity for reflection and deepening. The American psychotherapist and writer Thomas Moore suggests that the disempowerment we may feel when we are ill may serve a purpose.

> Weakness has its own rewards. As it becomes less literally a trait of personality and more a quality of soul, its many forms transmute into more subtle virtues such as vulnerability, openness, the capacity to feel and to be affected, flexibility and compassion. (1990, p. 153)

Freud's aim of changing neurotic misery into ordinary unhappiness will not necessarily persuade an insurance company to part with its funding. It may not get people back to work as might a course of medication. Nevertheless successful psychotherapy can facilitate the transformation of depression and anxiety into energising anger and reflective sadness. Research into negative moods done at the University of New South Wales concludes that sadness promotes "information-processing strategies best suited to dealing with more-demanding situations" (Lehrer, 2010). When we are aware of what we need and have the energy to act, meaningful change can happen. We can then thank the symptom for providing both the necessity and the opportunity for change.

The metaphorical body

The psyche can be thought of as the "inner" life of the body. This is not meant in a literal way such as we might understand that the brain and nervous system are located inside the body. Rather we mean that the psyche can be understood to be the body as it is lived and experienced from within. The body can be seen as the embodiment of the psyche. In giving our attention to the body and its symptoms, we can sometimes overlook the fact that the body and its symptoms are not just physical. They are also metaphorical. When we describe a problem as a "headache", suffer a "pain in the neck", need to take a "painful step" or are "sick" of some circumstance, we intuitively grasp this fact. Sometimes symptoms can point to psychological issues that lie behind them.

We use the word "metaphor" to describe something that "carries us beyond". In the case of the relationship of the body to the psyche the metaphor can carry our attention beyond the literal physical symptoms to the emotional, psychological, and spiritual concerns which sometimes underlie them. In psychotherapy we can recognise both the opportunity presented by a symptom and catch something of its unconscious significance by regarding it in a metaphorical way.

Let us take for example an instance of a young married woman. Whilst neither she nor her husband considered themselves to be in an "open marriage" they both engaged in repeated extra marital affairs and one night stands. Often these were a way of expressing anger and of equalising the power balance between them by "paying back" the partner. Neither partner seemed able to get to the root of this hurtful pattern. In the course of therapy she developed a severe ear infection. It was accompanied by a dream which in turn revived a forgotten memory. In her dream her mother was whispering into her ear. She recalled that as a child her mother would sometimes use her as a confidante describing her secret illicit extra marital affairs. She had "forgotten" this and disassociated herself from these memories. As the memories surfaced into consciousness in the context of her psychotherapy she was able to take action that led to improvements in her circumstances.

Another instance would be the case of a good looking, golden haired, blue eyed young man. He was an only child who grew up to be the "apple of his mother's eye". In his twenties he was a charmer and seducer of women, but as he entered his thirties he wanted a more committed relationship. His insecurities and lack of emotional maturity made him incapable of achieving this. He was also a chronic sufferer of ulcerative colitis. As he explored his early years in psychotherapy he spoke of growing up in a household with his elderly disabled father slowly dying of bowel cancer whilst being nursed by his mother. His mother's love seemed to be conditional upon his being her beautiful "golden boy". As he got more in touch with his "shitty" feelings of insecurity and anger, the colitis condition greatly improved. He was able to reveal and own these unattractive parts of his nature and find a greater degree of self-acceptance which in turn enabled him to enter more deeply into relationship.

In these cases we can see that the power of psychotherapeutic attending to the metaphor represents a deeper resolution and a more profound degree of healing than would a course of antibiotics. It is worth noting too that both the symptom and the dream are perfectly natural occurrences. Psychotherapy "attends" or pays attention to such natural healing processes allowing them to more effectively achieve their ends in a culture that dismisses the importance of dreams and suppresses symptoms.

Psychotherapists who work in depth will agree that that which is suppressed and disowned does not go away. The writers Dethlefsen and Dahlke chart the "degrees of escalation" by which psychological issues become progressively more deeply imbedded in the body.

1. Psychological phenomena (thoughts, wishes, fantasies).
2. Functional disturbances.
3. Acute physical disturbances (inflammations, wounds, minor accidents).
4. Chronic conditions.
5. Incurable processes, physical changes, cancer.
6. Death (through illness or accident).
7. Congenital deformities and conditions (karma) (1991, p. 85).

We can see that in first case referred to above the symptom of the infection emerged from the third level of escalation. In the second case the condition was more at the fourth level. Symptoms are the key by which we may gain access to what is being suppressed. According to this model the more we suppress our symptoms the more deeply embodied they will become. Or to put it another way; if we are deaf to the symptom which starts as a whisper (say a wish, a thought, a fantasy, or a dream) it may become the shout of a chronic organic condition that cannot be ignored. At this stage we may have little option other than to become locked into a battle between medicine and disease. Psychotherapeutic healing aims to work in depth with the natural energies of the embodied psyche. The symptom is a welcome ally in this task.

A deeper kind of healing

As health practitioners we need to be able to recognise and appreciate the nature of health or wholeness when we encounter it. In order to facilitate healing or "wholing" we need to do our best to understand the processes by which deeper, more comprehensive levels of health can be attained. Let us look further at how the experience of illness can be understood as a part of health.

Consider the case of Paul, a man in his fifties. He spent the whole of his working life in a caring profession working for low pay. He enjoyed the human contact and appreciated the emotional rewards of working with his vulnerable and appreciative client group. He chose this career path despite the best advice of his father. He also chose it despite being trained and having a talent for a much more lucrative job in industry. He was lately promoted to a better paid administrative role. He felt it necessary at that stage to sacrifice his client work and take on the new role on in order to secure a better retirement package.

Paul considered himself to be inadequate and felt unable to meet the demands of his domineering female manager. He didn't complain. He judged himself to be "too slow" and felt he should be doing all he could to deliver what was expected of him. For some months he had been using beta blockers prescribed by his doctor to control his mounting anxiety. He further medicated himself by drinking too much and would sleep through most of the day when he was not at work. Unbeknownst to his boss he would sometimes sneak into work on Saturdays in order catch up with his demanding work load.

Eventually he cracked. He suffered panic attacks, emotional outbursts, and exhaustion. He then considered himself to be "ill". His doctor said he needed time away from work. He came to psychotherapy in the hope that he might learn how to be rid of his symptoms and cope more successfully with his life.

Physician, psychotherapist, and patient will all agree that this client is "ill". But when did he become ill? Would we agree with him that his illness began on the day that he became incapable of work due to his incapacitating symptoms? Did it begin when he first used beta blockers to control his anxiety? Or was it on the day he accepted a promotion to a less emotionally rewarding but better paid desk job? Did it begin when he abandoned his potential career in industry? Or did the illness begin at a time he can scarcely remember and in circumstances that he can no longer fully recall?

How will he or we know if and when his health has been restored? Will it be when his symptoms are less and he can resume his work role? For a time he was able to feel less anxious and fulfil his duties thanks to his prescription for beta blockers. Did this treatment improve or damage his health?

Counsellors and psychotherapists in the UK are sometimes asked to assess the success of their interventions by a before and after questionnaire such as the Generalised Anxiety Disorder or "GAD"—7 standardised rating scale. Has the client more or fewer symptoms as a result of the treatment? How does the improvement compare with the relief offered by CBT, SSRIs, Pregabalin, Benzodiazepines, etc.? Medical wisdom has it that treatment success is best measured by the speed and degree of symptom relief.

In the case above the symptoms proved to be a gateway to deeper and more profound issues than how best to reduce stress or deal more effectively with a bullying insensitive manager.

Paul reflected that it was not only his oppressive boss that he desired to please and felt un-entitled to confront. He had also been married for many years to a woman who exploited him financially. She owned her own home and rented it for a private personal income while he paid the whole of the mortgage for their joint home. The couple had no children together and both had incomes. Upon separation she demanded, and was legally entitled to, half of the value of this home. It was as if he gravitated into relationships with exploitative domineering women and felt unable and un-entitled to protect himself.

Further reflection uncovered shameful personal and family secrets. He was a child in a large family. As early as the age of seven he sensed that there were secrets and tensions between his father and his sisters. As a young man these feelings became focused when two of his sisters revealed that they had been sexually abused by his father. At the time his mother was unaware of these goings on. He suspected that she chose to ignore what was happening because she felt overburdened by the demands of the large family. He wondered if perhaps she willingly overlooked what was happening in order to be relieved of his dad's attentions. She made light of the sisters' revelations by saying it was "all in the past" and best not dwelt upon. He wondered if Mum was in fact correct. Perhaps it really was a bad idea to rake over these painful issues from the past in therapy.

Paul later made the painful revelation that he too had in indulged in "sexual play" with the sisters. He felt he was therefore in no position to judge his dad negatively when he had done the "same thing". He was deeply ashamed and remorseful about this. In fact it seemed that much of his adult experience made a new sense in the context of his background. He had rejected his father's materialistic values and chosen a career that focused on service to vulnerable people. He allowed himself to be bullied and exploited by women as though in repentance for his misdeeds as an adolescent.

Psychotherapy enabled him to explore these issues in depth and begin to alter lifelong patterns. He could see the bigger picture or larger context of which his behaviours were a part. It opened the prospect of a deeper healing or "wholing" of his issues and increased self-awareness and realisation. In fact we could say that there was a sense in which his problems and patterns were not strictly "his". He had imitated, as children do, the behaviours of his parents. In a sense he had "inherited" a dysfunctional family pattern. When he ended this behaviour as a young adult he had only partially broken away from the pattern. It was partial in the sense that it appears to have been an overcompensation governed by shame and guilt. Therapy afforded the opportunity to find a deeper level of healing. The symptom relief he attained in the form of lessened anxiety was merely a by-product of a much more profound and transformative change.

It is possible also to speculate that if his father had been the client in therapy, he too would have had a story to tell that would put his behaviours into a context. Perhaps the family pattern extended back for many generations. Perhaps the true origins of Paul's illness began long before he was even born. We are reminded of the Biblical verse wherein God is said to "punish the children for the sins of the fathers to the third and fourth generations" (*Bible*, 1970, p. 202). His family story would of course be set in the context of the broader social issues of the time. In this way healing at depth is not just a personal healing. It heals also at a family, social, and even perhaps at an ecological level. The task of a therapy that works in depth can be transformative both personally and socially. Such therapy owes a debt of gratitude to the insistent demands of the symptom which, if it is not suppressed or disowned, can serve the function of keeping the work on course.

Serious organic disease as an agent of healing

Let us briefly take a look at a second case that illustrates this principle and involves a severe organic complaint; one which threatened the possibility of death.

A man in his forties worked as in international lorry driver. He suffered a stroke and was obliged to give up his work. He suffered partial paralysis on one side of his body and a lost the power of speech. He was however given the opportunity to attend a day centre for stroke sufferers. There he managed over the course of a little more than a year to regain his physical mobility and linguistic ability. To achieve this he was forced by circumstances to confront both his physical and emotional vulnerability. He learned to communicate deeply with other stroke survivors. Part of his rehabilitation involved art therapy. He discovered that he had an outstanding talent and was later able to sell his art works to help support the organisation that facilitated his recovery. Despite his recovery he chose not to return to his life on the road.

In a case like this we can see that even a life threatening organic condition such as a stroke can perform a healing or wholing function. The loss, the limitations, and the disabilities suffered by this patient are plain and obvious. It requires time, perception, and thought to recognise that the illness also provides certain opportunities. This self-reliant man in the prime of his life was accustomed to thundering down the autobahns and motorways of Europe, crossing national frontiers in a powerful forty tonne articulated lorry. Suddenly he found himself being pushed by others in a wheelchair. After an initial period of depression he was forced to admit and to confront his vulnerability. He learned to acknowledge and express his need for the help of others. It is not the case that he suddenly *became* vulnerable and needful. All human beings are subject to death, illness, and injury. All of us have physical and emotional needs and dependencies at all times whatever our outward circumstances.

The stroke performed the role of forcing him to become aware of these underlying and unconscious realities. He was in time able to marshal his resources and learn to see the humanity in others who like him were disabled. He developed a greater capacity for empathy. This was a quality that was not especially needed in his former lifestyle. He developed also the power to express himself in art and discovered a dormant and neglected side of his nature. By the time he had recovered from his stroke he had become more "whole". He had achieved a fuller degree of self-realisation. He had by necessity learned the art of "patience" as a result of being a patient. Some learning in life requires time and the force of necessity in order to become fully realised. It is as though our fate is determined at another level of consciousness beneath and beyond that of the conscious ego. This consciousness is beyond the personal and can be considered "objective". Illness, even life threatening illness, can be a means by which we are healed and become more whole.

Normality and order

Medicine and those psychotherapeutic approaches most favoured by medicine measure their success by symptom removal and the restoration of "normal" or "orderly" functioning in life. This can be at the cost of deeper healing. We can see in the first case above that the client's attempt to maintain his normal orderly functioning with the medical assistance of beta blockers served to block rather than to facilitate a deeper healing. If his symptoms can be thought to have had a meaning or an intention, it would be to draw his attention to underlying unresolved issues that required his conscious awareness in order to restore his health.

Psychotherapy holds the view that the psyche has an underlying tendency to strive toward a fuller realisation by means of drawing the attention of the conscious ego to unresolved issues via the symptom. This is sometimes referred to as the "self-actualising tendency" or as "individuation". If we too readily label and identify symptoms as psychiatric disorders we can overlook the deeper healing energies of the psyche. Psychological "order" can then mean adaptation and adjustment to an external environment that itself may be disordered and in need of healing. A client who is empowered by the knowledge of his or her own needs and requirements for healthier living may be able to alter or abandon an unhealthy environment. In the above case of Paul, in addition to his in-depth work on his "inner" world he was able to better his circumstances by leaving the oppressive workplace.

When we closely examine symptoms with a view to identifying both physical and psychological disorders there is a danger of overreaction. It is estimated for instance that in scanning for physical abnormalities with a total body scanner that the average person will have some twenty-five abnormalities without any signs of illness whatsoever (Hegde, 2006, p. 139). Similarly a browse through the *Diagnostic and Statistical Manual* (DSM) might cause us to wonder whether we have signs of disorders with such acronyms as ADHD, OCD, MDD, GAD, PTSD, PmDD, BDD, SAD, BPD, TD, FTD; or eating disorders, and personality disorders. If so there is a corresponding list of pharmaceutical medications and short term solution focused therapies with which we can combat these symptoms. It is notable that in the United States public billboard advertising will draw our attention to the possibility that we may have "disorders" such as Attention Deficit Hyperactivity Disorder (ADHD) without even knowing it. We are encouraged to self-diagnose in order that we might enjoy the benefits of medication.

The metaphor of combat

> A murderous array of disease has to be fought against, and the battle is not a battle for the sluggard [...] I steadily investigate the disease [...] and I proceed straight ahead, and in full confidence, towards its annihilation. (1848, p. 33)
>
> Thomas Sydenham,
> (the "English Hippocrates") 1624–1689

When we are faced with acute and deadly diseases that require immediate attention we will of course quite rightly assemble all of our resources in order to survive. The medical community sometimes describes this response as a declaration of "war" on certain of these diseases. The British Department of Health for example speaks of a "war on heart disease". Under the presidency of Richard Nixon the United States declared a "war on cancer" which continues to be funded at a rate of five billion US dollars a year. When we enlist the metaphor of war, combat, and battle there is unlikely to be the kind of inquiry, patient forbearance, and understanding that might lead to a deeper healing. While this may be justified in a crisis, it wastes what may also be an opportunity for growth and wholeness such as we saw in the second case example above.

The combat metaphor wears particularly thin when we apply it to non-deadly conditions such as the common cold. The British pharmaceutical company GlaxoSmithKline for instance advertises their Beechams brand with such slogans as "Fight back against colds and flu", "The enemy and us", "The power to fight back". What we are encouraged to fight back against are, of course, the body's natural means of healing and of eliminating toxins. Common cold and flu symptoms are not the illness. They are the healing. The sweats, the phlegm, the diarrhoea, the coughs, the fatigue are all there for a very good reason. The body demands that we take a step back from our normal routines in order to restore and recuperate. Instead we "fight back" by doing what we can to carry on as normal and block the processes of toxin elimination.

Once again this is no small scale battle. Americans spend some three and a half billion dollars annually on over the counter remedies for coughs and colds. This is despite the fact that most colds clear up naturally in about a week without treatment of any sort. By comparison the USA spent less than a billion dollars on the 2011 Libyan intervention.

Psychotherapy that works with the forces of self-realisation, self-actualisation, and individuation needs to attend to the underlying requirements of the psyche. Labelling and the suppression of symptoms are on the whole unhelpful in this kind of work.

Actual psychotherapy

We have noted that the medical world is more interested in the signs of disease than it is in symptoms that do not point to an identifiable underlying biological problem or physical disorder. The signs of disease point to verifiable underlying physical conditions that can be measured and corroborated. These can then be addressed by the medical professions with their array of drugs, surgery, and other tangible interventions that have been proven to be effective. Symptoms that do not indicate an underlying physical condition have less interest and are considered to have less relevance to the practice of medicine.

A condition such as chronic fatigue syndrome or myalgic encephalomyelitis (ME) for example is not widely recognised or accepted as having an underlying medical cause; nor are there specific treatments. In some cases the symptoms may be regarded as signs that point to an underlying medical condition such as an underactive thyroid. When this and other explanations are eliminated the diagnosis of "chronic fatigue syndrome" or CFS is given. If this is the case the usual prescribed treatment consists of medications that address its symptoms such as painkillers and antidepressants.

We have seen too that a condition such as bipolar disorder is responsive to psychiatric medication in the form of lithium. Exactly how and why the medication is effective remains unknown. The psychiatric response to this condition does not identify or address an underlying illness. It modifies a symptom.

We have also seen that research indicates that depression may be associated with lower than average serotonin levels. A lower than average level of serotonin however does not necessarily indicate a state of depression. Depression cannot be explained as a biochemical phenomenon on this basis. The symptom stubbornly remains a symptom. It is not a sign pointing to an organic condition that lies beyond itself. Its true significance remains unknown.

If we were to use the combat metaphor favoured by many medical campaigners, we could say that medicine "employs an arsenal of weapons" to "fight off" and suppress unpleasant symptoms of which it does not fully, if at all, understand the cause. Because there are no known biological causes such conditions are often regarded as psychosomatic and are believed to have their origins in the psyche rather than in the body. Their cause lies "beyond the pale" as it were; in the unruly realms beyond reason or governance of the conventional and prevailing view of health.

Our work as psychotherapists, or as attendants to psyche, demands that we do not attempt to arm the government (ego) to fight off the terrorists (the illness). Nor do we arm the freedom fighters (the illness) to overthrow the oppressive dictatorship (ego). We are there as honest brokers attempting to mediate the conflict. We try to remain emotionally present and responsive but un-invested in either side of the dilemma with which we are confronted. By hearing the needs that are being presented by both the ego of the patient/client and by the split off aspect of the psyche which is embodied in the symptom or illness we may be able to create an atmosphere of healing. We can loan emotional support, foster connections, and offer conceptual frameworks that may help to ease the dis-ease and move a step closer to wholeness or health.

Of course there is understandably much skepticism when it comes to the point of listening to the voice of an illness and tending to its needs. Few people actively want to suffer. Sufferers are eager to find an underlying physical cause which can be alleviated and ideally removed. If this can be done effortlessly by means of a medication that has no noticeable side effects so much the better. Many patients and clients long for a treatment that can get to the root of the problem and remove it. Far from recognising an opportunity to expand self-awareness and find a healthier more fulfilling way to conduct their lives, patients very often resent what can feel like the inferior status of an illness that has been wholly or partially attributed to a psychological origin. Psychosomatic illness can be felt as a humiliation. It can seem to be a slur on the character of the sufferer. It is regarded as an "imaginary" illness that can come tainted with the stigma of self-indulgence, malingering, and avoiding the challenges of life. The anxious, the depressed, and the chronically fatigued are not necessarily taken as seriously or accorded the same degree of empathy and regard as are those with diseases that are attributed to physical causes.

Conversely, we are not surprised if physical illness affects the patient's psychological wellbeing. The symptom is then understood as a sign or consequence of a "genuine" physical condition and therefore it can excuse and justify the patient's suffering. So obvious is it to us that our physical state will affect the psyche that we don't feel the need to have a word for somato-psychic illnesses; or illnesses which are based in the body but which affect the psyche. Of course we will feel emotionally unwell if we are physically sick. And if we don't we might well be regarded as admirable heroic "survivors". In contrast the idea that a purely psychological condition affects our physical health comes with a tinge of shame. It is hardly surprising that patients can seek the security of a proper hard medical diagnosis. When working in a half-way house for mental health sufferers, I can recall how residents who merely had the diagnosis of "personality disorder" would return from their doctors in stress and despair. They sought the much more serious and in effect "prestigious" diagnosis of "schizophrenia" or "manic depressive mood disorder". Who would take them seriously if they didn't have a proper medical diagnosis which explained and justified their symptoms?

Many believe that illness is fundamentally either physical or psychological. It is either out there where it can be objectively measured and observed or it is in the invisible psychological realm where its origins can only be indirectly viewed. In reality psyche and soma are not two separate domains but are two aspects of the same thing. We could even argue along with Jung that the psyche is the more basic and fundamental of these two aspects of our being because "we know matter only in so far as we perceive psychic images mediated by the senses" (1958, p. 12). Our medical tradition remains very largely entrenched in the Cartesian divide between a substantive objective outer reality and an invisible subjective inner world.

Some patients feel that what mainstream medicine can offer in the way of treatments for such psychosomatic illnesses is insufficient. They may turn to psychologically orientated treatments such as cognitive behavioural therapy (CBT) which enjoys a measure of public approval and funding largely because it happily speaks the language of demonstrable quantifiable improvements in terms of symptom relief. We have seen that in terms of symptom reduction its results can be shown to compare favourably with those offered by drug treatments and by long term psychotherapy. However none of these approaches seem to fare an awful lot better than placebo.

There are some sufferers who seek more than symptom relief and look for what we might call "actual" psychotherapy in the sense of the "wholing" or healing that we have been discussing. We aim to actively "attend to soul" in the etymological sense that defines the root meaning of the word psychotherapy. We aim to actually "do" the activity that the word we use for our profession indicates that we do. In this case the symptom is not something to be overcome, eliminated, or suppressed. We consider it to be the voice of an aspect of the psyche of which we are either unconscious or insufficiently conscious.

We can think of symptoms as parts of our potential psychic being that are not connected with ego consciousness. Symptoms and indeed disease itself may hold the energy of aspects of consciousness that have been disowned, suppressed, or repressed. In this case they may need to be re-membered or taken back into consciousness. The collaboration of a psychotherapist can loan support and offer conceptual frameworks to make this possible. There may also be aspects of consciousness which are in a state of emergence which cannot yet be recognised if our conceptual structures are too limited.

Also it may be that the heart is not yet strong, mature, or educated enough to embrace the emotional charge that lies behind the symptom. In psychotherapy the education of the heart is every bit as important as is that of the intellect. A sufficiently aware, mature, and emotionally healthy psychotherapist may also be able to facilitate this process. In either case it is the voice of something unknown that insists on intruding into the prevailing consciousness. We have explored the fact that psychotherapy is much more than is recognised by its medical definition as "a set of techniques". Gone from most trainings are the intensive three to five times weekly training analytical sessions that lasted for a period of years. The profession's increasing tendency to shift psychotherapy trainings into university settings and to award academic degrees tips the balance of attention toward the academic, the technical, and the conceptual.

Unlike a medical approach in which the doctor treats the patient in an attempt to restore wellbeing, in psychotherapy we enter a collaborative process. Psychotherapist and client work together. The joint task is to find ways to allow the energy within the symptom to be felt and heard more clearly. If this approach is successful the result may well include the lessening or ending of the presenting symptoms. However we can regard this as a by-product rather than the focus of psychotherapeutic work.

The success of this work is not to be measured by symptom relief alone. This can be achieved by drugs and other therapies that suppress, dissociate, and disconnect the intrusive energy behind the symptom. From psychotherapy's perspective these results can be regarded as counter therapeutic. Success can instead be recognised by the alterations in consciousness that occur when connections are made. There is a broadening and deepening that occurs when consciousness connects with the inner life of the symptom. This is not recognised by the feedback questionnaires beloved of psychotherapy's institutional funders. It is instead a felt body sense; a feeling of "aha", a sense of homecoming, a sense of realising and recognising what at some deeper level we knew all along. This experience is the true measure of psychotherapeutic success. It is in fact the very definition of "integrity" which at root means "virginal" or "untouched". It is a recollection of an initial untouched psychological state from which we have become estranged. This can take the form of a reconnection with something that has been forgotten, suppressed, or repressed; a literal re-membering of a part of the traumatically dis-membered psyche.

We noted from Dethlefsen and Dahlke's work that even deeply embodied physical disease will contain psychic content. Healing may potentially happen on a psychological level even if the body is too damaged to recover physically. There is such a thing as a healthy way to live with an illness. Ultimately there is also the possibility and hope of a "healthy" death. Death is the one guaranteed certainty for all living beings. It is a hard concept for medics to grasp. I once discovered this when addressing a group of medical students. I posed them the question "Is there such a thing as a healthy death?" This apparently bizarre question seemed to flummox the group. There was a period of seemingly baffled and bewildered silence after which one young man tentatively offered this suggestion. "Well, I suppose if someone were young and fit and they were hit by a bus and killed, then maybe you could say that it was a healthy death." The student was clearly thinking in accord with the World Health Organisation's definition of "complete physical, mental, and social well-being". Illness was being seen as the opposite of health. As psychotherapists I propose that we respectfully beg to differ.

We may need to consider the possibility that forgotten, suppressed, repressed, or never consciously known aspects of the psyche continue to have a life of their own. This life of the symptom and the disease may lie outside either our personal or our collective awareness. It is not just individuals who have psychological blind spots or areas that need development in order to adapt to a changing environment. Cultures do too. Arguably our scientifically based technological culture is in desperate need of renewed awareness of the power of the imagination when it comes to matters of health.

We have seen how in terms of psychotherapy the relevant questions are, "What does the illness want?" "What are the symptoms saying?" "What is my response to these unavoidable demands of the psyche?" This is fundamental to the whole ethos of the profession. If illness is a voice of the psyche then there is no way that psychotherapy can comply with medicine's demand to fight against it. We cannot make an enemy of illness or its symptoms. Our best hope is to make an ally of the energy behind the symptom. Given our own emotional and conceptual limitations along with the limitations of the culture of which we are a part success cannot be guaranteed. We cannot be satisfied by simply helping to restore a sense of wellbeing and fostering a return to normal functioning. If psychotherapy attempts to make this its aim there is a corresponding loss of soul. We are left with what Jung called "psychology without the psyche". His observation of 1933 remains relevant today; "And so it comes about that all modern 'psychologies without the psyche' are studies of consciousness which ignore the existence of unconscious psychic life" (1933, p. 206).

Psychotherapy's aim is to give the unlived life that has become embodied in the symptom or the illness a chance to express itself. Jung says of illness that:

> We do not cure it—it cures us. A man is ill, but the illness is nature's attempt to heal him. From the illness itself we can learn so much for our recovery, and what the neurotic flings away as absolutely worthless contains the true gold we should never have found elsewhere. (1964, p. 170)

Georg Groddeck, who many consider to be the father of psychosomatic medicine, says the same thing slightly differently. He says that to actually cure an illness and relieve a symptom would be:

> [...] to correctly interpret that which this totality is trying to express through symptoms and to teach us a less painful mode of self-expression. (Ramos, 2004, p. 40)

Abraham Maslow raises the question

> Does sickness mean having symptoms? I maintain now that sickness might consist of not having symptoms when you should. Does health mean being symptom free? I deny it. (1968, p. 7)

He maintains that we are sometimes healthier when we appear to be sick than we are when we appear to be healthy.

Taking inspiration from Jung, Maslow, and Groddeck we can recall that the word "heal" in its etymological root sense means "to make whole". It then becomes clear that only some medical approaches and some forms of psychotherapy actively pursue this objective. Our question must be how best do we enable and facilitate "healing". As psychotherapists we must wish that the patient or client either develops a healthy relationship with their illness or emerges from it as a more complete human being.

CHAPTER FOUR

The origins of Western medicine

Clinical: adj. 3. scientifically detached; strictly objective.

—*Makins*, 1979, p. 304

Let us now look at the roots of Western medicine. This takes us back to a time when the line between what we now regard as the realm of psychotherapy and that of medicine was less clearly drawn. We discover a very different approach to health which was based on a different way of experiencing the world. We also discover something of great insight and value that has been lost to the practice of modern mainstream medicine

Hippocrates

Western scientific medicine traces its origins to Hippocrates. Some call him the "father" of modern medicine. He lived some two and a half thousand years ago on the island of Kos in Greece and is referred to in the writings of Plato. Hippocrates is credited with initiating an ethical and rational style of medicine which believed that "health and illness follow a pattern which can be understood through careful observation"

(King, 2001, p. 17). Hippocratic medicine is rational, logical, and considered. The writings of Hippocrates and his followers include theory and observation of specific diseases and detailed case notes of treatments. The writings stress that "nothing is random" and they urge the doctor to "overlook nothing". They emphasise that nature itself is the ultimate healer; "Nature is the physician in disease." The continuing influence of Hippocrates is recognised today by those medics who choose to take the Hippocratic Oath. The oath invokes and swears by the old Greek gods with particular reference to Asklepios, the Greek god of healing (Hart, 2000, p. 222).

Without contradiction the objective, observant, and rational Hippocrates also considered himself to be, in a spiritual sense, a "son of the god Asklepios" or Asklepiad. If we regard Hippocrates as the "father" of our modern medicine, then it follows in this metaphorical sense that Asklepios is the "grandfather". Hippocrates practised his art in what we can perhaps best describe as a state run hospital that was free of charge to the patient (Kerényi, 1959, p. 51). As this hospital later developed, it took on the full role of a healing temple sacred to Asklepios, known as an Asklepion. The Hippocratic approach was a part of a much larger picture. Doctors or "Asklepiadai" saw themselves not only as skilled observers and prescribers of therapies and medicine, but also as the servants of the god Asklepios. It was considered that Asklepios did the work of healing with the assistance of his Asklepiadai. There was less danger at this time that doctors might become heroic or grandiose. Healing was seen as a divine art performed in humility as a service to and on behalf of the god.

Impediments to understanding

These ancient Greek origins have been officially recognised and celebrated by the medical profession since the mid seventeenth century (Schouten, 1967, p. 128). At this time the "rod and serpent" of Asklepios began to be chosen as an emblem of the medical profession. The image takes us back to a time when the mind functioned in ways so radically different to those of the present era that it is extremely hard for us to imagine or grasp. There are at least two major hurdles to overcome in order to gain some hint or flavour of this state of mind. We first need to try to imagine how it felt to live in a time before René Descartes. Descartes taught us that there is a strict and unbridgeable divide between the mind and matter or between objective facts and subjective fantasies. Although particle physicists are today seeing things differently, it is fair to say that in the Western world at least; this is an almost universally held assumption about the nature of reality. Out of respect for our ancient ancestors, this assumption must be set aside if we wish to feel some sense of empathy for their views. We must be open to the possibility that our perspective may simply be a "different" one rather than the "right" perspective. We must try to image ourselves into a frame of mind in which the divide between inner and outer realities is less absolute. In this state of mind intense and powerful "inner" realities could be perceived as though they were outer realities. It is a condition of mind that we today most often associate with diminished cognitive ability such as might occur in altered mental states induced by drugs, fatigue, or illness; or attribute to tribal peoples or children. This was not necessarily the case in the ancient world when heroic Greek figures such as Odysseus and Theseus were said to have conversed with gods.

We must be prepared to recognise that at base, scientific objectivity and what we call the "clinical" perspective are mental constructs which we have acquired over the course of the centuries. They can sometimes be effectively employed in the service of healing. However scientific objectivity does not always aid healing. Healing does not necessarily require science or objectivity. Living bodies have healed themselves successfully for as long as our planet is old.

We have a second major obstacle to gaining an insight into the mindset at the time of the origins of Western medicine. This is to understand the implications of the great paradigm shift from polytheism to monotheism. This occurred around two millennia ago together with the rise of the Christian religion. We need to be able to imagine our way into a polytheistic mindset that apprehended truths as multiple rather than as singular. Rational and mystical religious approaches were practised side by side in Asklepieia or healing temples of the ancient world. Both paradigms were considered to be true in a way that it can be difficult for the contemporary mind to comprehend (Hart, 2000, p. 136). It is not so much that two parallel but incomplete and contradictory truths were held side by side. It was more the case that two or any number of truths could all simultaneously be absolutely true without contradiction. The Hindu scholar Professor Max Müller described the polytheistic view in this way.

> When these individual gods are invoked, they are not conceived as limited by the rank and power of the others, as superior or inferior in rank. Each god, to the mind of the supplicants, is as good as all the gods. He is felt at the time as a real divinity, as supreme and absolute, in spite of the limitations which, to our mind, a plurality of gods must, entail on every single god. (Wilkins, 1882, p. 11)

In accord with this view the polytheist might agree with the Christian or Jew that there is indeed a single supreme and absolute god. At the same time, much to a monotheist's likely frustration and incomprehension, they would regard this god of supremacy and absoluteness as but one of the panoply of gods. Bearing these considerations in mind let us think about the origins of Western medicine.

The two sides of medicine

Who is this figure to whom Hippocrates and even today many physicians continue to swear an oath? Asklepios is first referred to as a historical figure in Homer's *Iliad* written in 800 BCE (Homer, 1969, p. 59). Asklepios was a renowned healer and a ruler of Thessaly who lived five centuries earlier than this in around 1300 BCE. His two sons Machaon and Podalirios served as physicians in the Trojan War. Machaon is said to have specialised in manifestly physical illnesses and injuries while his brother Podalirios focused on "invisible" illnesses. Together they encompassed both the inner and outer aspects of healing.

We can see here how from the earliest recorded times the Greeks seemed to hold a balanced view of healing as an art that required attention to both the visible, manifest aspects of healing and to the invisible inner realms. In the two sons of Asklepios we can recognise two sides of the healing process. These are the visible and the invisible aspects; or we could say the physical and the psychological. Western medicine has of course made great strides in the visible side of medicine. Microscopes, x-rays, magnetic resonance imaging (MRI) scanners, etc., bring more and more previously invisible conditions into the visible realm where they can be addressed in the manner familiar to Machaon. To gain the attention and respect of a medical tradition that follows largely in the wake of Machaon, some look to brain scans, genetics, and blood chemistry analysis in an attempt to bring psychological matters into the visible realm. Failing access to hard science we are apt to provide quasi scientific, quasi physical statistical evidence such as generalised anxiety disorder (GAD) and patient health questionnaire (PHQ) scores. Whether brain activity can be thought to be the cause or the result of psychic activity is a moot point. Identifiable causes for what we call psychiatric illness remain stubbornly hard to identify. There remains today no known organic cause for such common conditions as schizophrenia, depression, bi-polar mood disorder, etc. The genetic and chemical aspects that are present in such conditions can equally well be present in those who suffer no symptoms of psychiatric illness at all. We must conclude that the psychic and the physical, the invisible and the visible are two sides of the same process which can best be thought of as a kind of feedback system.

Psychotherapy can be regarded as a mode of healing in the invisible realm in the manner of Podalirios. Arguably our role as psychotherapists demands that instead of investigating the physical basis of psychological illness we need to approach things from the other equal and opposite direction. We need to explore the psychological basis of physical illness. Psychotherapy is an art that addresses the other half of the task of medicine. This side of illness has been relatively neglected and in many cases ignored by the modern Western medical tradition. In the Greek tradition both sides received equal recognition and respect as is evidenced by the roles of Asklepios's two heroic sons in the Iliad.

Asklepios

In mythology Asklepios was understood to be a son of Apollo. Amongst Apollo's many attributes he was the god of light and the sun, harmony, order and reason, truth and prophecy, healing and plague, music, and poetry. Asklepios was the son of Apollo's union with the mortal princess called Koronis. We can recognise here a precursor to the Christian myth of the god of light who fathers a child by a mortal woman and who will later go on to be a friend and saviour of humanity. Myths vary as to whether Koronis was unfaithful to Apollo and provoked his murderous wrath or whether she died in childbirth. In either case Asklepios needed to be cut from his mother's womb, whereupon Apollo entrusted his care to Kheiron or Chiron the Centaur.

A centaur was a mythical creature said to have had the body of a horse joined to the torso of a man. Kheiron was believed to have passed on his learning in the ancient traditional medical arts to the young Asklepios.

Some commentators have speculated that this mythical creature might actually refer to the last of the Neanderthals who some believe may have still survived at this time by removing themselves to "remote and hilly country where they were often seen riding shaggy ponies, their hairy bodies indistinguishable from their mounts" (Houston, 1987, p. 8). Viewed in this way it can be seen that the figure of Asklepios brings together the natural healing methods of Kheiron with the light and reason based philosophies of Apollo.

The staff and serpent of Asklepios

Physicians in ancient Greece were itinerants. They walked from town to town in order to deal with the sick. When Asklepios is depicted or represented in statuary he is shown with his walking staff. At the most obvious level this symbolises his ability to be where he is needed and when he is needed (Edelstein, 1945, p. 229). In a more symbolic sense the staff can be understood to represent his reliability, his supportive helpfulness and his wisdom. However in some representations the staff is shown less as a walking aid than as the rough branch of a tree. The branch is sometimes shown still carrying a few leaves. In this case we may see it as a metaphor for the primal vegetative life force of nature with its potential for re-growth. It acknowledges and celebrates those mysterious forces which rise up from the dark underworld to facilitate healing.

The Asklepian staff is clearly meant to indicate more than simply the wandering life of the ancient Greek physician. The symbolic nature of the staff is reinforced by the fact that it is encircled by a rising serpent. In the ancient world the serpent was already a familiar image for healing. Its history goes back at least until 1800 BCE when it is referred to in the Sumerian epic poem of Gilgamesh, one of the world's earliest surviving literary works. Nigizzida was the son of the Mesopotamian God Ninazu (whose name meant "Lord Physician"). Nigizzida's symbol was a rod with two entwined serpents (Patton, 2009, p. 12).

The ancients believed that snakes had the knowledge of healing. The serpent was considered to be sharp sighted, vigilant, faithful, and wise. In the gospel of Matthew for example we are urged to "be wise as serpents and harmless as doves" (Bible, 1946, p. 9). Snakes also have the apparent power to renew themselves by shedding their skins. The fact that snakes slither on their bellies and generally make their homes underground associates them with the element of earth. Their tunnels were thought to provide them with access to the subterranean gods; while their lack of visible genitalia was taken as a sign of their supreme creative powers (Hart, 2000, p. 41). We can see then that in both the image of the staff and in that of the serpent, Asklepios has to hand the primal chthonic regenerative powers of the both the animal and vegetable kingdoms. Although he is the son of Apollo, the god of light and reason, he draws equal strength and power from the mysterious dark unconscious elements.

It is curious that the chosen symbol for contemporary medicine should honour the dark, the mysterious, and the natural in ways that are hard to reconcile with modern technological and pharmaceutically orientated health care. It is easy to associate the modern hospital with the Apollonic qualities of bright light, reason, and precision. It is harder to see how this can be united with the dark and mysterious elements of healing such as were practised in the ancient world at the time when Western medicine first emerged. Of course many medics are unaware of the history and associations that lie behind the emblem of their profession. An example of this is the case of a general practitioner who was in psychotherapy at the time of his retirement. Upon hearing a reference to the rod and serpent he was convinced that he had never seen nor heard of such a symbol. He needed to go home to his wife and to check his letterheads to be convinced that this image had indeed accompanied him throughout the whole of his medical career.

As well as being forgetful, modern medicine is apparently sometimes also confused as to exactly which ancient Greek god it is honouring. Instead of the rod and serpent of Asklepios some medical and medically related institutions use the caduceus as their symbol. This is especially so in the United States. The caduceus is a rod that is crowned by a pair of wings with two serpents coiling up on either side of it. It is the emblem of the god Hermes (or Mercury). One survey found that sixty-two per cent of professional healthcare associations used the rod of Asklepios as their symbol while in the commercial health care sector seventy-six per cent of organisations used the Caduceus symbol (Friedlander, 1992, p. 78). Hermes was a messenger of the gods. He was regarded a patron of boundaries and travellers. Amongst other persons and qualities in his domain he was a protector of weights and measures, commerce, orators, and thieves.

The founding of the Asklepieia

The figure of Asklepios evolved from a historical figure to that of a hero god and finally to full status as an Olympian god (Hart, 2000, p. 17). However, unlike the other Olympians Asklepios was neither aloof nor prone to vengeance. In statuary his facial expression was often shown to convey intense inner emotion as though in the words of one commentator, "he is assailed [...] by the sufferings of men, which it is his vocation to assuage" (Kerénye, 1959 p. 23). It is evident that Asklepios was a precursor and model for the later figure of Christ. Asklepios died after incurring the wrath of Hades (the god of the underworld) after he raised the dead. He gave his life in the service of suffering humanity and was known by his supplicants as a "saviour". His cult lasted well into the Christian era until the fifth century when the church, holding that "the true Saviour a jealous god" (Edelstein, 1945 p. 256) ordered that his temples and sanctuaries be destroyed.

In the early classical period great healing centres and temple complexes were built to promote healing and to honour Asklepios. At a time when Rome was being ravaged by an uncontrolled epidemic Asklepios was brought by sea with much ceremony to that city believed to be incarnated in the form of a sacred snake. There a great temple and sanctuary built in the shape of a boat was devoted to him on an island in the Tiber. Today a modern hospital stands on the site testifying in a very literal way to the sense in which modern medicine is built on Asklepian foundations. The supreme act of healing was once accomplished by communion with the god Asklepios in a dream state. Today an area of glass floor leading to the diagnostic imaging department reveals the underlying foundations of the Asklepion temple. A chapel devoted to St. Bartholomew was built over the temple of Asklepios. This associated Bartholomew with medicine as is reflected today in the name of St. Bartholomew's (or St. Bart's) research and teaching hospital in London.

The Romans spread the Asklepios cult throughout the empire. This included remote and far flung outposts such as Britannia. Representations of Asklepios and votive offerings for cures can be found at sites such as Bath, Chichester, Lydney, and other locations throughout England, Wales, and parts of Scotland.

Healing in the Asklepion

Because Asklepios was deeply connected to the healing power of the underworld, it was considered important to build temples and healing centres where he could reside and where his presence would be more strongly felt. The healing power of Asklepios could be more fully known in temples dedicated to his worship and in the company of his priests and of fellow sufferers in need of healing. The principal healing centres or Asklepieia in Greece were located at Epidaurus, Trikala, Kos, and Pergamum (in what is now Turkey).

Like a modern hospital the Asklepieia provided all that could be offered in terms of a rational and considered approach to healing based on careful observation and study. However in a way that is not characteristic of a modern hospital, a healing environment was considered to be an essential requirement for the recovery of health. Such sites were not necessarily chosen for ease of access as is the case in the modern world. Indeed a contemplative pilgrimage or journey of intent along with the personal sacrifices and inconveniences this held for the sufferer was considered to be a part of the healing process. In order to maximise the likelihood of successful healing, sites of inspiring natural beauty were favoured. The writer Henry Miller describes the inspiration he felt as he travelled through an "idyllic landscape" on his approach to the Asklepion of Epidaurus.

> It is sheer perfection, as in Mozart's music [...] the road to Epidaurus is like the road to creation. One stops searching. One grows silent, stilled by the hush of mysterious beginnings. If one could speak one would become melodious [...]. The landscape does not recede, it installs itself in the open places of the heart. (1941, p. 80)

Miller clearly responded to the landscape in the way desired and intended by the creators of the Asklepion. Above the entrance to the Asklepion of Epidaurus was a magnificent marble archway inscribed with the words:

> Pure must be he who enters the fragrant temple, Purity means to think nothing but holy thoughts. (Edelstein, 1945, p. 164)

We can imagine something like a hospital, combined with a modern health spa, contained within a spiritual retreat. The Asklepieia provided a wholesome move away from the pathogenic circumstances of the sufferers of illness. A well situated site would be able to offer fresh air and a plentiful supply of spring water with special healing properties. In keeping with the chthonic nature of Asklepios springs were regarded as a means by which the visible and conscious everyday human world was healed and refreshed by the powers of the gods of the underworld. Psychotherapists who work in depth will recognise the healing potential of this movement of energy up from the dark underworld into the light of consciousness. Additionally a plentiful supply of water was needed for bathing, ritual cleansing, and hydrotherapy. Careful attention was also given to diet and physical exercise. All of these factors were regarded as necessary in order to summons and to mobilise the body's capacity for healing.

Nonetheless healing and illness were believed to require more than attending to the needs of the physical body. Social, emotional, and spiritual dimensions were also addressed. One means by which the social and emotional elements were attended to was by providing opportunities for collective catharsis in the theatre. The theatre in the Epidaurus Asklepion remains today a remarkable monument and an impressive architectural achievement. It bears testament to the sophistication and importance of these healing centres. This theatre is capable of accommodating 15,000 spectators with acoustics so good that it remains possible today for the entire audience to hear a coin that is dropped at centre stage.

A performance at the theatre would be designed to arouse and evoke emotion. As a member of the audience you would be taken beyond the limited confines of your ailing and conflicted ego. Audience members would hold on to one another and join together in vocal response to the dramas that were unfolded before them by the likes of Aeschylus or the playwright Epicharmos whose thirty-five dramas acclaimed by Plato have been lost to history. Intense cathartic drama would act both as a kind of group therapy and would help to release withheld and unconscious emotions. Once again this would bring the hidden dark sacred serpentine underworld energies into conjunction with the clear bright light of Apollo. The god Asklepios himself would personify the harmonious reconciliation of these energies.

After the intense high drama unrefined energies would also be evoked and welcomed by what American author and philosopher Jean Houston describes as the "wild and woolly satyr plays—ribald, rascally comedies often featuring men dressed in goatskins bopping each other over the heads with six foot phalluses—and this elevates your spirits" (1987, p. 5). Then would follow the comedies intended to lighten the heart and enlist the healing power of laughter.

In addition to its physical beauty the site would dazzle the senses with some of the most magnificent art, statuary, and architecture of the age. Houston evocatively and poetically imagines it like this:

> [...] you walk down the streets of Epidaurus where you see marble temples blazing with color, beautiful paintings of the lives of the gods and heroes, and sculptures whose haunting harmonies speak of the godded human and the humanised god—dedicated to the Asclepian by the great artists of the day, Praxiteles, Phidias, Polygnotis. Your eyes quickened and your senses stimulated, you sight sacred street processions going by—stately files of priests, hymning Apollo; drumming, dancing ecstatics devoted to the cult of Dionysius waving ivy-covered wands, chanting worshipers of Aphrodite bearing an ancient wooden icon of the goddess. This prompts you to enter the temples of the gods—the Olympian gods and the lesser gods as well—where you pray and invoke their powers. (1987, p. 4)

Attention was directed to the gods, or in more modern terms those archetypal powers and energies which are common to us all. These energies course through us and take us beyond the ego. Supplicants were encouraged to recognise that there were deep mysterious forces at work. These could not be fully understood or controlled. If in today's world the gods have become diseases as Jung believed, the Greeks encouraged a respectful surrender to this bigger picture. This lessened the likelihood that the stubborn demanding ego would block the wholing or healing process that was demanded by the god through the illness. Unlike a modern hospital, the Asklepieia did not accept pilgrims whom the physicians/priests considered to be facing immanent death. Nor did they accept women who were about to give birth. The atmosphere would thus be free of the disturbing stress inducing sounds and activities associated with birth and death. The belief that death could not enter the sacred precincts would have greatly reassured and comforted patients. The focus would instead be more readily fixed on the hope and expectation of cure and renewal.

Dream incubation

After a period of this physical and psychological purging and purification the physician priests would determine when a suppliant was "clean" enough both mentally and physically to be ready to enter the "abaton" or "place not to be entered unbidden". Here a direct encounter with the god Asklepios himself was expected. This was achieved by a night time ritual which involved the supplicants being ritually dressed in white. Priests then led them into the dimly lit temple of Asklepios where they would encounter marble stelae and tablets that were donated by the grateful recipients of healings. Inspired by the possibility of such healing they would approach the more than life sized statue of the god with a dog lying beside him. Both of these would be surrounded by the living sacred temple snakes. These were a type of non-venomous European tree snake known as the *zamenis longissimus* that can grow up to six feet in length. Here they would make an offering of honey cakes to the serpents and make a sacrifice to Asklepios as they requested a healing.

The culmination of the stay at the Asklepion was the ritual temple sleep or "incubation". The sufferers would be invited into the dimly lit, incense filled, sleeping area of the abaton. Here they would sleep on a couch or *kliné* as it was known in Greek with the expectation of experiencing a healing dream. This would take the form of a personal encounter with the god himself, either in human form or in the form of one of his sacred animals as serpent or dog. In one of these forms Asklepios himself would either grant a cure outright or prescribe a remedy. Should none of these images appear in the incubated dream the priests would interpret it as best they could and prescribe treatments based on the imagery and their medical knowledge. During the night the priests and priestesses dressed as Asklepios and his daughters Hygeia (health/cleanliness) and Panacea (all healing) would attend to the sleeping people accompanied by the temple dogs and snakes. While the incubants slept they would gently apply salves and ointments while the dogs would lick the wounds and the snakes would slither about amongst them. After this period of intense psychological and physical cleansing in the extraordinary environment of the Asklepion we can imagine how the weird and disorientating atmosphere of the abaton might well help to engender an exceptional dream.

In the morning those patients who had been healed would celebrate and shout their praise and thanks to Asklepios. Some patients would likely feel that they had been successfully healed. Others would feel that their condition had greatly improved. Those who had not been healed or had not seen a dream would be told to continue to remain at the Asklepion and return to the abaton until they too had received a dream.

After such healing, payment was due; though the poor were subsidised. This would take the form of money according to the means of the pilgrim. Additionally, sacrifices and thank offerings were presented to the god. This might take the form of a votive offering representing the body part that had been afflicted. These are commonly to be found on the sites of Asklepieia all over the ancient world including Britain. Sometimes the healed patient would compose a paean or song of praise to Asklepios or erect a stone stele describing their cure which would inspire other sufferers in search of healing. Sometimes the wealthy would contribute a bas-relief or low relief stone carved picture depicting their cure. This would embellish the beauty of the temple. The traditional animal sacrifice was the cock. The dying wish of Socrates was that a cock should be sacrificed on his behalf to honour Asklepios.

Without doubt the personal encounter with the god as he appeared in a dream was central to a treatment at the Asklepion. It should not be imagined however that the prescribed treatments were therefore of a strictly mystical or psychological nature. Prescriptions were more likely to come from the sunlit, rational, Apollonic side of the nature of the god. Treatments prescribed in the Asklepieia would include the use of drugs, hypnotherapy, exercise regimes, hydrotherapy, and laying on of hands. More surprisingly perhaps surgical interventions were quite common. Cancers for example were known to be treated by burning (which could be seen as a primitive form of radiotherapy) or cutting tumours from the body (Walton, 1979, p. 60). This is referred to in the work of Hippocratic physicians as long ago as the fifth century BCE (Papavramidou, 2010, pp. 665–667). Most important of all however was considered to be a positive and calming environment.

The tradition of Asklepios today

The tradition of Asklepios did not die with the destruction of the temples under the reign of the Emperor Constantine the Great in the fourth century. Particularly in the Eastern Orthodox Christian tradition elements have survived right through to the present day. We have noted how the figure of Christ embodies many of the qualities of his predecessor Asklepios. These include his mix of divine and human parentage, his blameless life, his heroic deeds on behalf of humankind, his teachings of love and compassion, his extraordinary healing powers that enabled him even to raise the dead, and his ultimate sacrifice and later resurrection as a divinity. Moreover, the convention of portraying Jesus as the familiar long haired bearded figure we know today did not begin until after the destruction of the Asklepian healing sanctuaries. Prior to this time Jesus was depicted as a beardless and often shorthaired youth. He acquired these attributes of Asklepios only after the end of polytheism and Christianisation of Rome and Byzantium.

Physical healing through dreams still occurs in certain churches in the Eastern Mediterranean. Twentieth century silver anatomical thank offerings can be seen today in the chapel of Saints Kosmos and Damian near to the site of the Asklepion of Corinth. While on the island of Tinos in the Aegean the Church of the Panagia Evangelistria is a centre for miraculous healings proffered by the Patron Saint of Greece "Our Lady of Good Tidings". A local nun named Sister Pelagia was guided in a series of visions to unearth a lost wonder working holy icon. This icon is thought to be the work of the Apostle and Evangelist Luke. The icon was indeed found amidst the ruins of a long buried fourth century chapel dating back to the time of the destruction of the Asklepian temples. As was the case with the Asklepieia the chapel was situated beside a healing spring. Healings are attributed to the icon which is the most venerated of all icons in Greece. The church now hosts massive pilgrimages. Votive offerings for successful healings are displayed amongst a dazzling mass of gold and silver offerings inside the church. These include a golden plaque offered by King Constantine of Greece in 1915 offered in gratitude for his recovery from a life threatening condition (McLees, 2000, p. 42).

Outside of Greece other modern healing shrines such as that at St. Winifred's holy well in Flintsire in Wales and Lourdes bear many features that carry the characteristics of the old Asklepieia. Jessica Hausner's 2010 ambiguous semi-documentary film entitled *Lourdes* contains a sequence in which the main character receives a healing dream and is able then to leave her wheelchair.

Today the Asklepion snake remains strictly confined to the logo of modern medical practice. However hospitals today are witnessing the return of Asklepios's other sacred animal—the dog. In the UK today there are over four and a half thousand "pets as therapy" (PAT) dogs. These animals bring comfort and healing to hospital patients as they visit nearly seven million bedsides in the course of a year. Today the healing power of the dog is also being reenlisted in the form of the "psychiatric service dog". These dogs offer aid in the healing of ex-service personnel. They are trained to recognise the signs of psychiatric disturbance such as paranoia and hallucinations. They can interrupt repetitive and injurious behaviour and do such things as remind their owners to take their medications, retrieve objects, guide their owners from stressful situations, and act as a brace should they become dizzy. Near Los Angeles, a centre offers effective treatment for young people with behavioural problems based on interaction with wolfdogs i.e. dogs of various breeds that have been interbred with wolves.

It is interesting and somewhat ironic to note that our modern words *"clinic"* and its adjective *"clinical"* are derived from the Greek *kliné* as used to denote the couch of the sacred healing dream about which we have spoken. Even at the very core of modern medicine's most heroic efforts to remain "scientifically detached" and "strictly objective" (Makins, 1979, p. 304) is a tacit acknowledgement of medicine's long forgotten deep mysterious spiritual roots. Not until the turn of the twentieth century did the couch of the healing dream reappear in medical practice in its new form as Freud's psychoanalysis.

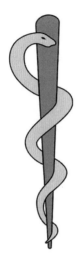

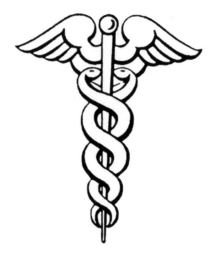

The Rod and Serpent of Asklepios.   The Caduceus of Hermes.

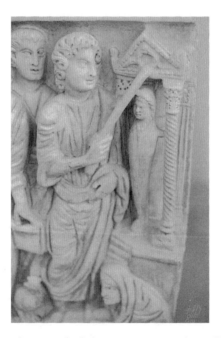

Early Roman sarcophagus relief showing a young beardless Christ raising Lazarus from the dead with a magic wand.

CHAPTER FIVE

Apart from or a part of?

We have seen that etymologically speaking, the psyche may be thought to be the soul or the breath. This notion of the soul once led Jung to question, "Why has the self created the body? I don't know why we are not wind; we might be forms made of air and beyond sex or appetites" (1935, p. 120). In order to explore this idea let us now consider something of the nature of the ancient Greek psyche. How might a Greek at the time of the Asklepieia have experienced the world? We have reason to suppose that their common assumptions about the nature of reality and the way they felt about being embodied and ensouled were radically different to ours.

Imagine, if you can, inhabiting a body in which you feel as if your thoughts arise near to your heart and not in your head. You experience your mind as being in your chest. You think about that which is close to your heart. You think with your body. Perhaps if you wish to voice your thoughts you breathe out and allow your thoughts to escape from your lips in the form of words. If you should choose not to voice your thought your breath will still escape. It is the subtle moisture of your breath that then conveys your unvoiced thought into the world. All of those who breathe in the air around you inhale the atmosphere of the thought of your heart; be it voiced or unvoiced. All are influenced. The unspoken thought still goes into the world where it becomes a part of others.

Imagine too that every inhalation takes in the atmosphere that has been built up by the voiced and unvoiced thoughts of others. With each breath you take on board a little of the atmosphere created by others. These most subtle of vapours feed your lungs with what others both wish and do not wish to convey. These vapours that were believed to be inhaled and exhaled with each breath were known in the Greek language as "atmos". The sphere in which the atmos of all breathing things exist was known as the "atmosphere".

Every person you encounter, every animal, and every plant is breathing. These too exchange their essences with you and build an atmosphere; an atmosphere that is composed not just of gases but also of thoughts and feelings. Imagine if you can, that what you see and what you hear are also the subtle breaths of your surroundings. Like a fine vapour, sound and vision enter through your ears and eyes. These receptive senses also breathe in the world about you. These vapours too are taken in as they are breathed down into your lungs.

These fine breaths of atmos condense inside your lungs and are stored in your body. Your brain, your spinal cord, and the marrow of your bones hold the moisture of these essences. This supply of the breathed in thought of the hearts and essences of the world is your intelligence. Your intelligence is none other than the intelligence of the world about you. The more of this "sap" that you contain, the more "sapient" you are. Likewise your contribution to the breath of the world as but one of the planet's many homo sapiens plays its part in adding to the intelligence of the world and in making the world what it is.

Every breath is a communion with the world. Everything makes a difference. There is no withholding. There is no resisting the influence of the environment. Nor can you withhold your participation in the world as it is experienced by others.

Classical scholars provide evidence to suggest that such may have been the sense of self we may have had in the days of ancient Greece (Onians, 1951, pp. 66–83). This was a time when the psyche was understood to be the breath. Each of us partook in the breath of the world.

It is calculated that each breath we take comprises approximately ten sextillion atoms (ten to the twenty-second power) (Murchie, 1979, p. 320). Each breath we take will contain atoms that have been breathed by anyone living on the planet that we care to name. Because the atmosphere is a finite resource it will also contain atoms that have been breathed by any historical figure you care to name whether it be that of your remotest ancestor, of Jesus Christ, or Genghis Khan. Similarly as a part of the community of animals we quite literally breathe in the material that sustained the family pet of childhood, the mammoth, the sabre toothed tiger, and the dinosaur. Part of the physical fabric of these ancient beings of the past is right here and right now built into the structure of the body that you inhabit.

In this way we can see that what the Greeks called psyche (the breath) is indeed shared. It is in a state of perpetual exchange with the environment. Jung's view was that we are in the psyche. The psyche is not in us.

The same can be said of the body. The body which we inhabit is not separate from the body of the world. In addition to the air we breathe, the food which has built and sustained our bodies during our lifetime comes from nowhere other than the living world around us. A healthy human body is not self-sustaining and independent. Microbial cells in and on the human body outnumber human cells by a ratio of ten to one (Wenner, 2007). The waste products of the digestive tract and of the kidneys, the shedding of skin, perspiration, hair, and nails all enter the living environment where they in turn sustain further generations of living beings. If we so choose we can think of our bodies as self-contained and separate from the world; but perhaps our bodies can be more accurately thought to have something of the nature of a whirl-wind or a vortex that circulates the already existing materials of the world in a consistent pattern. Our pumping hearts and bodily processes circulate these materials of the living world of which we are but a frag-ment. They create a recognisable and familiar form. We proprietarily call this form "me".

Albert Einstein expressed his understanding of this sense of our commonly felt alienation and separation from the universe in this way;

> A human being is a part of the whole, called by us "Universe",
> a part limited in time and space. He experiences himself, his
> thoughts and feelings as something separate from the rest—a kind
> of optical delusion of his consciousness. (Calaprice, 1950, p. 206)

Each breath confirms that we are in a state of perpetual interchange with our surroundings. The writer David Abram draws attention to the fact that we commonly refer to what we take to be the obvious fact that human beings live "on" the earth (2010, p. 100). There is the earth and then there is us living upon it; separate entities in relation to one another. It is actually far more accurate to say that we live "in" the earth. The atmosphere which we breathe is a part of the physicality of the planet. Along with the oceans and land masses it too turns with the rest of the planet. If this were not the case we would be subjected to constant westerly winds of 1000 miles per hour. We live in the earth of which the atmosphere is a part as fishes live in the water. We are, as it were, a feature of the atmosphere and physicality of the planet.

We can feel ourselves to be intimate not just with the world but with the cosmos. Science tells us that the most basic building blocks of life are atoms which were formed in the stars during the origin of the universe. These have combined in myriad ways over the aeons of geological history. We know of three and a half billion years of the evolution of life which have cooked these chemicals into ever more complex living forms. In the womb we review the history of evolution. The human foetus lives in the saline waters of the womb and in its early development it has gills. The blood retains the salinity and temperature of the primal seas from which life is thought first to have emerged onto the land.

When we look at human cultural development we discover a similar pattern. The self is a composite of the collective. Our oldest hunting, foraging, and survival skills were probably learned from the animals with which we shared and share our world. Some Native American tribal lore regards the human being as the "little brother" of the animals. In this tradition we are not thought to be the apex of evolution but instead are considered to be the junior partner of the animal kingdom. We are the newcomers; the vulnerable creature who in terms of sustainable living has yet much to learn in comparison with the wisdom of the animals. We are indebted to our teachers.

With the emergence of language we can again see how our individual identities are assembled from the pre-existing conditions of tradition and cultural word usage. In this sense the dead never die. They live in and through us. We use the words, expressions, and frames of reference that were expedient to them even though we may have long since forgotten that to which they refer. By and large this is not a problem.

While there are many thousands of examples which could serve to illustrate this point, for now let us ask what we are really saying when we say "by and large" meaning "on the whole" or "all things considered". Do we know that in a sense we are hearing with the ear of and giving voice to the commonly used terms of reference of the seventeenth century mariners in our collective ancestry? A "large" wind blows in the direction of travel. "By", on the other hand, refers to sailing into the wind. A ship that can easily sail with or against the wind makes good progress "by and large".

There are diverse hosts of such persons who speak though us. They generally command only the most minimal of awareness from the speaker. The dead speak through our voices not only in their choice of turns of phrase and frames of reference. Their choice of words also displays their attitudes, perspectives, and psychological issues. Modern psychotherapy can confirm what has been known since Biblical times; that the sins of the fathers are visited on their children "to the third and fourth generation" (1970, p. 160). Those who partake in depth psychological work will be aware of family patterns that perpetuate themselves through us unless and until they are challenged and altered in the light of conscious awareness. This, by the way, is the true meaning of the Halloween "trick or treat" custom. Our ancestors live on inside us. These invisible presences can sometimes "trick" us. Their perspectives may no longer relate to the world as it is today; just as they may conversely hold a needed wisdom that we have lost. They can haunt and complicate our lives until we recognise them and their autonomy. We can then give them the "treat" of our critical attention and/or the appreciation that they require. We are at that point enabled to get into relationship with the ghosts of our ancestors, just as we do with our biological parents. In both cases this can sometimes be done with the help of psychotherapy. Otherwise we can be prone to re-enacting their issues. We can in effect be "possessed" by them in the form of their often archaic and ill adapted attitudes and values.

The bioenergetic psychotherapist John Conger puts it this way:

> Not only are we left as children with our parents' unlived lives skulking in the shadows, their unresolved dilemmas, but we are unconsciously caught in their world view and their assumptions about every aspect of reality. We are caught in a subjective bubble, a projected, inherited universe a closed system, seeking solutions to problems that defeated our parents and using only the tools they have prescribed. If education is valued by a family member, then education becomes the over-determined source of answers. If

money is valued, money becomes the solution. Rigidly doing the opposite of what we saw or was expected of us is of course, to be as deeply ensnared as our compliant siblings. Tragedy and severe conflict may be the only means to tear the envelope of inherited fantasy fashioned around us. (1994, p. 120)

We are accustomed to laying personal claim to the thoughts and impulses that occupy our minds. Indeed to suggest anything other than this can conjure up frightening visions of madness. Yet language, education, and culture are all acquired from without. We furnish our minds with thoughts in a comparable way to how we might select the furniture in our homes. These are predominantly pre-made products. They are arranged and cared for according to our own tastes and temperament.

The ancients understood things differently. In Egypt for example thoughts were regarded as invisible entities somewhat akin to birds. They might flutter through our minds of their own volition. We might or might not choose to capture them, to cage them, perhaps to let them sing for us, but they were not ours in the way we regard them in today's world. The maxim "Don't believe everything that you think" has a salutary wisdom. Our thoughts are like guests in our house. We may invite them in and entertain them for a while during our fleeting lifespans but they are not ours. They have their own life with their own history and their own destiny. We need to relate to our thoughts rather than identify and merge with them. The thoughts we have but don't know we have, have us. We could say that thoughts make excellent servants but poor masters.

C. G. Jung encountered this during a spontanious visualisation in which he discovered "Philemon", an autonomous "imaginal" being which he regarded as his inner guide. As we discussed earlier we choose the word imaginal here in order to distinguish this from deprecating term "imaginary" which carries connotations of something unreal which is invented by the conscious ego. The figure said that he, C. G. Jung:

> [...] treated thoughts as if [he] generated them [him]self, but in his view thoughts were like animals in the forest, or people in a room, or birds in the air, and added, "If you should see people in a room, you would not think that you had made those people, or that you were responsible for them." It was he who taught me psychic objectivity, the reality of the psyche. (1961, p. 176)

Jung thus discovered what he called the "objective psyche". This is the idea that thoughts must first be objectively perceived. We recognise this autonomy of thinking when we say that a thought "occurs" to us. It is the thought that is the active party when it presents itself to us. We do not command it. When this happens thoughts can be entertained, rejected, or "owned" in the sense that we may wish to claim as our domestic property any artefact or creature that we find in the environment about us. Jung understood that there was something in him "that (he did) not know and (did) not intend, things which may even be directed against (him)". Consequent to these insights we can say that "my thought is mine" in a comparable way to the way a caged bird may be "mine". Otherwise there is a danger it may be we who find ourselves in the cage; caged in by the limiting thoughts and concepts with which we have identified ourselves rather than be liberated and enlightened by them.

Jung had rediscovered something that would have been easily accepted by the Greek psyche. To the Greeks dreams were objectively "seen" rather than subjectively "had" as we would say. The dream for the Greeks was not a subjective experience but an objective one. But for us it is clear that Jung's idea of an objective psyche stretches and confounds the very notion of what is normally understood by the terms subject and object. Collins English Dictionary defines the word "subject" as "that which thinks or feels as opposed to the object of thinking and feeling".

But what happens when our thoughts and feelings themselves become the objects of our thoughts and feelings? What then do we think and feel about what we find ourselves thinking and feeling? Psychotherapy can invite us to stand back and observe those thoughts and feelings with which we occupy our minds. From that base we are then in a position to judge the nature of our inner dialogue. To some extent we can then choose how to modify it with a view to creating an enhanced sense of wellbeing.

As we witness these we must ask if we generate our own thoughts and feelings or are they produced unconsciously by processes we do not fully understand? Are involuntary and perhaps unwanted thoughts and feelings triggered or even created by others such as parents, spouses, society, or ancestors? It is not uncommon for people to say "you made me feel ..." as though they were not responsible for their own state of mind. Is it more accurate to say, as does Jung, that we merely perceive our thoughts and feelings? Then, as we have discussed, we may respond *to* them whilst being aware that we are not responsible *for* them. To perceive and to re-evaluate our thoughts and feelings in the light of consciousness is essential to psychotherapy.

Depending on how deeply we are able or willing to go in this self-examination we can enter a deeper state of awareness as we become conscious of the thoughts and feelings we use as the criteria by which to evaluate and judge the thoughts and feelings we discover. We ask ourselves from what perspective are we examining and evaluating our thoughts and feelings? With what values do we decide how best to relate to our thoughts and feelings? Is our self exploration determined for example by the shallow ego centred core values of a technique like cognitive behavioural therapy (CBT)?; namely being goal orientated, problem focused and time limited? Or from a Greek perspective; to what god are we aligned? Through the eyes of what deity do we see?

If we are unconsciously aligned with a particular archetypal perspective or a "god" as the Greeks might have understood it we are in a sense "possessed" by that perspective. Fundamentalisms of every order whether they are religious or rationalistic reveal an inability to see through other eyes than those with which they are identified. If *we* are right then it follows that *they* must be wrong. In the words of former US president George W. Bush "you are either with us or you're with the enemy". There is only one truth. We can develop a godlike sense of omniscience when we do not recognise the archetypal view or god through whose eyes we see. We might speculate that the psychological benefits of recognising a plurality of gods or archetypes is that it enables us to dis-identify from a viewpoint with which we might otherwise unconsciously identify ourselves. Simultaneously it helps us to recognise the truth and validity of other modes of experiencing and viewpoints. The humility and ritual demanded in sacrifice or tribute to the god safeguards that we stay in a conscious relationship to those archetypal psychic energies rather than become unconsciously possessed by them. In this sense we can see that this ancient polytheistic psyche has a certain psychological sophistication and articulation that we as modern-day rationalists lack.

We have discussed the etymological sense in which psychotherapists are attendants to the psyche or soul. We have seen how in the Greek understanding the soul is built from the environmental "atmos" or subtle vapours in the breath. Our essential being is a distillation of environmental elements. That which is without becomes that which is within, that which is within becomes that which is without; ebbing and flowing with each breath. We are each an absolute and inalienable part of the world. We cannot exist apart from it.

As psychotherapists we pay "attention" to and "attend" to the soul. It is the soul, that subtle entity that is simultaneously both me and a quality of the world around me that does the work of healing in psychotherapy. It is not just the work of the therapist or even of the client. The client in modern psychotherapy is in some respects like the supplicant to the god. The client must humbly acknowledge that their problems and issues are beyond their present power or ability to resolve. He or she must travel to the place of healing and there become a "patient" willing to "patiently" sacrifice both time and money to attend psychotherapy. Both parties need to acknowledge that it is not the psychotherapist who leads the healing process and brings the transformation. It is the soul or the god itself. Need we remind ourselves that the psychotherapist is not a god but is merely an attendant of the soul? There are some psychotherapists who proudly boast of their skills and of the effectiveness of their innovative techniques to evoke profound and rapid transformations in their clients. We might suppose that such practitioners lack this sense and perception of being in service to a greater force than they. Without this perception we are in danger of ego inflation and hubris.

Interbeing

Let us consider further this unfamiliar, strange, and paradoxical idea that something of our very essence can be understood to be simultaneously both within us and outside of us in the world. How can we understand the nature of the relationship of the inner to the outer if not through our Cartesian consciousness? Thich Nhat Hahn is a Vietnamese Zen Buddhist monk who has coined the word "interbeing" to describe his understanding of this view. He puts it simply:

> If you are a poet, you will see that there is a cloud floating in this sheet of paper. Without a cloud, there will be no rain; without rain, the trees cannot grow; and without trees we cannot make paper. The cloud is essential for the paper to exist. If the cloud is not here, the sheet of paper cannot be here either. So we can say that the cloud and the paper "inter-are". (Hahn, 1988, p. 9)

He continues to elaborate the theme to show how without sunlight neither the tree nor the cloud can be and how human beings and culture are essential to creation of paper and are therefore implicitly within the sheet of paper. If the sun should cease to shine or the rain to fall, or the logger to work, or if the factory were to close, then the piece of paper would cease to exist. If any of these non-paper elements were to return to its source the paper could not be. If we look deeply enough with an intuitive eye we can see this truth implicitly within this or indeed within any phenomenon including that of our own being.

To ground this idea he developed a structured meditation practice so that it may be felt and known experientially. By spending time focusing and concentrating on each of the elements as they are experienced both within and outside the body it becomes possible to sense more deeply the continuum between our personal existence and the existence of the world about us. We become more grounded in a non-Cartesian way of experiencing. We get nearer to what the existential psychiatrist R. D. Laing described when he said, "My experience is not inside my head. My experience of this room is out there in the room" (1967, pp. 18–19). The meditation practice can help us to realise the obvious truth that we are not separate from the world. Laing stressed the fact that, "My psyche is my experience, my experience is my psyche." Thich Naht Hahn says:

> The sun is just as necessary for our bodies as our hearts are. The forest is just as necessary for our bodies as are our lungs. Our bodies need the river as much as they need our blood. If we continue to meditate like this we shall see that we can let go of the boundaries between "I" and "not I" and thus we can overcome the distinction between birth and death [...]. (Hahn, 1993, p. 48)

Not in the world but of it

As well as dealing with our Cartesian assumptions about the nature of our experiences, we are also impeded from this kind of understanding by the legacy of our Christian heritage. In the Gospel of John, Jesus is reported to have said "I am not of the world" (1946, p. 106). Later we are exhorted:

> Do not love the world or the things in the world. If anyone loves the world, love for the Father is not in him. For all that is in the world,

the lust of the flesh and the lust of the eyes and the pride of life, is
not the Father but is of the world. And the world passes away, and
the lust of it; but he who does the will of God abides forever. (1946,
p. 222)

Such verses as these can be, and are, interpreted by scholars in a number of ways but they clearly raise issues when we attempt to understand
our relationship to the world in which we live our lives. We can easily remain fearfully entrenched in a sense of separation and alienation
from the environment. The view offered by Thich Nhat Hahn promises
a transcendent realisation and liberation to be had from an appreciation
of the true nature of our relationship to the world. The Christian view,
at least on the surface of it, suggests the opposite of this. It seems to fall
into dualism by driving a wedge between the life of the incorporeal
spirit and that of the world.

The green man

If the Christian tradition can lead to difficulties in appreciating the
nature of our connection to the living world around us, another figure which is commonly found in the churches of Britain and parts of
Europe takes us in a very different direction. Largely ignored, disre-
garded, and misunderstood, this persistent figure too is a part of our
heritage. Often hidden away out of obvious sight either on the interior
or exterior decoration of many of our churches and cathedrals, as well
as on some state buildings such as the British Houses of Parliament,
is an enigmatic figure known as the green man. This figure is often
to be found in the cornicing among gargoyles or on decorated col-
umns. It may be carved into the woodwork of pews or above door-
ways. The figure has many variations but it usually depicts a man's
face made either of a single leaf or of a number leaves. There are two
eyes, a nose and a mouth. Sometimes the mouth is shown to be spew-
ing out vegetation.

Despite the fact that this figure is often found in churches it is not
considered to have any Christian significance. It is in fact a far more universal and ancient archetypal image. It can be recognised in the Islamic
tradition as the figure of Khidr or the "Green One" who guides souls on
the spiritual path. It harkens back also to the Pagan worship of northern Europe. The leaves are reminiscent of the woodland glades where
the old gods were worshipped in the days when northern Europe was

mostly forested and where religious rites were performed out of doors. A similar likeness to the green man can be seen in the Celtic horned god of the animals known as Cernunnos.

In the iconography of ancient Egypt the green man can be recognised as Osiris who was the green skinned god of vegetation and of the underworld. Like Asklepios, Osiris can be considered to be another precursor to the figure of Jesus. Amongst his many other epithets he was known in Egypt as the "Lord of Lords", "King of Kings", and the "Good Shepherd". He was considered to be a god-man who suffered, died, and rose again to reign eternally in heaven. His faithful devotees believed they too would gain eternal life. His coming was announced by three wise men and his flesh was devoured in communion cakes of wheat which was regarded as the "plant of truth". Like the green vegetation itself Orisis died that he might be born again in the spring. By partaking in his flesh we unite with the life-giving powers of the earth and of the underworld (Walker, 1983, p. 749).

In the ancient Greek world that we have been discussing other aspects of the green man can be recognised in the goat-footed, pipe-playing god of the woodlands and of nature, known as Pan. He is also the god of the wild, of shepherds, flocks, and goats. He is often associated with sexuality. His name is in fact another word for no less than "everything". The Greek born writer Plutarch lived in Rome during the reign of the Emperor Tiberius in the first century of the Christian era. He wrote of a man called Thamus who was sailing from Greece to Italy. As he passed the Island of Paxi near Corfu he is said to have heard a divine voice calling from the shore. It said, "Thamus, are you there? When you reach Palodes, take care to proclaim that the great god Pan is dead" (Plutarch, 1936, pp. 347–501). When Thamus did this, the news was greeted from the shore with groans and laments." At the very birth of the Christian era the god of the woodlands and indeed of "everything" is said to have died.

Because the god Pan died at the advent of Christianity he can in some ways be seen as the antithesis of Christ. The archetypal psychologist James Hillman puts it this way:

> The death of one is the life of the other. The contrast appears in the symbolisation of their bodies, their geographies and their rhetorics. The one has the cave, the other the Mount; the one music, the other

Word; Pan's legs leap and dance, yet they are crooked, hairy, and goat-footed; Jesus' legs are broken and stretched, his feet crossed and nailed. Jesus the Good Shepherd; Pan, the obstreperous, unruly goat. Pan is naked and phallic; Jesus circumcised, covered and asexual. (2000, p. 8)

But of course the gods do not die any more than do the archetypes. They may disappear from conscious awareness but they do not die. In the case of Pan his likeness later reappeared in the popular Christian depiction of the Devil as the horned and cloven footed nemesis of Christ. It is worth remembering that Lucifer is of course imagined in the Bible as a bright angel whose name means "light bringing". Perhaps too the leafy, apparently innocuous, decorative and incidental figure of the green man that adorns our churches holds the memory and the connection to a power and a way of perceiving that to our cost we have long ignored.

Of course we as psychotherapists are very familiar with the fact that Pan is not dead. He is alive and well in the consulting room. He is spoken of frequently and regularly in psychotherapy practice in the guise of the panic attack. Panic gives us something of the flavour of the nature of this god or archetypal force when it has been neglected or ignored. In an insistent and undeniable way he does his essential work and calls us back to an encounter with our inner nature. When we are unconscious or out of touch with the energies that are carried by Pan we are subject to his attentions. What are the primal, sexual, animal, instinctual, unruly, impulses that are being denied? Are we at one with our own nature, our instinctual nature, the primary nature of being the particular human being that we are in the world? What impulses might arise in us that we would find hard to manage? With what conflicts might we wrestle if we dared to allow the energies of our deeper more authentic nature to course through us? What are the legitimate fears that are masked by and underlie the panic?

Straight from the goat

O goat-foot god of Arcady! This modern world has need of thee!

(Oscar Wilde, 1994, p. 125)

This is the dream of a twenty-seven year old outwardly successful married man called Jonathan who appeared to be coping well when for the first time in his life he suffered a panic attack. It was sufficiently severe to admit him into hospital as a victim of a suspected heart attack. After a series of tests and a night in the coronary care unit he was told that his condition was "only nerves". However, his panic attacks continued several times a day with such severity and persistence that they left him in an ongoing state of physical and psychological exhaustion. Over time he had become mostly housebound. His hypersensitivity was such that he became unable to tolerate bright lights, loud noises, or social interaction.

> I am sitting quietly in my room. Out of the corner of my eye I notice something like a folded paper Christmas ornament rolling about on the floor. As it rolls about it gets ever bigger until it is maybe six feet long. It stands on end and grows toward the window. I knock it down but it rises again.
>
> It turns into a big green paper man and talks with Rosa [his wife]. It tells her that he wants to be taken care of. The paper man sounds belligerent. Rosa agrees to cooperate and asks what we should do about visitors. Are we allowed to tell them about the paper man? He says he'd prefer it if visitors did not come to the house. I intervene and tell him he is being unreasonable.
>
> The paper man argues back and tells me that I am stupid. He says I don't know how to live properly. I am inauthentic. I need to be on my own because I care too much about the opinions of others and about owning things. I become angry at him. I insist this is not true. I agree that he is right insofar as I do sometimes care too much about these things but that if I feel this is the case, I always try to put it right. Although I make many mistakes what else can be done?
>
> The paper man seems to agree that I have a point. He now looks like a flesh and blood human being and closely resembles my male cousin. He suggests that we all call it a night. I feel we've reached an understanding. We embrace and I wake.

This impressive dream marked a turning point in what was becoming Jonathan's increasingly isolated and incapacitated life. His panic attacks had forced him to resign from a well-paid but highly pressured business job in the city that was both intellectually and emotionally unrewarding. He tried to cope with the stress of his job and his two hour commute each way to work by an increasing reliance on alcohol. His hypersensitivity forced him to reflect on his life as he was unable to take refuge in distractions such as television and superficial social interactions.

His anxiety state had stopped him in his tracks. It prevented him from pursuing the dangerous and unfulfilling path he was on. We can see from this point of view that the figure of the paper man in his dream represents a healing aspect that needed to emerge more fully into his consciousness. Over the course of the following months and years Jonathan was able to gradually reassemble his life on much more fulfilling lines. He developed his artistic talents and eventually retrained in more fulfilling work that involved caring for others. The panic attacks had destroyed his ability to live one kind of life and opened the opportunity to create another more healthy and sustainable lifestyle. Panic had delivered him to the coronary care unit. Jonathan needed to learn to care for and to live more from his heart in order to live in a more authentic way. According to the mythologist Barbara G. Walker the word panic "was originally the terrible cry of Pan who dispersed his enemies with a magic yell that filled them with fear and took away all their strength" (1983, p. 765). In this case we can see how "Pan" had frightened off and disempowered those forces with which Jonathan had on a conscious level become identified, yet which at the same time blocked his capacity to live in a deeper, more authentic, and fulfilling way.

If as healing professionals and as psychotherapists we can see beyond the presenting symptom; if we can recognise the archetypal forces (or gods) that underlie them, then maybe we can help to open a channel through which they make their way into conscious life and then, through the individual, into the world at large. At that point we perform a role which is something more akin to that of the Asklepiadai. We attend to, we pay attention to, we wait on, and we wait for those greater and deeper than personal forces that govern and underlie our conscious individual identities. We act as midwives to the soul and serve the gods. We value and welcome pathology knowing that the energy that lies within it potentially enables wholing or healing.

We can see here that the healing comes not from transcendence or rising above pathology. Nor does it come from the suppression or eradication of pathology. It is not a promise to be fulfilled in the next life in a better world to come. No, it comes straight from the goat; right here on earth and right now. It comes through pathology; from the insistent green intelligence of nature.

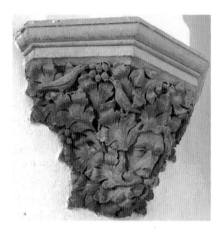

A green man carving from Sutton Benger church in Wiltshire, England.

CHAPTER SIX

The personal daimon

The myth of Er

The writer and mythologist Michael Meade describes soul (or psyche) as "the third element in the trinity of existence". He says that it fills the space between spirit and matter. It enables these opposites to remain related. It does this by grounding the spirit in the material world and by animating matter. Without soul or psyche we have the soulless Cartesian divide between dead inert matter and an abstract unworldly spirituality. He says that:

> When we lose our way in the world it is the soul's way of being in touch with the world that has been lost. We are most lost and truly abandoned when we have lost touch with our own soul, with our own inward style and way of being in the world. Soul is the missing ingredient when things fall apart, just as it was the animating ingredient that brought us to life. (2010, p. 119)

As we have seen, psychotherapy that attends to the soul is not best described as a set of techniques used to treat mental health and emotional problems with a view to alleviating distress. Rather it is the work of facilitating the soul's purpose and intent. It is as though what we are referring to as the soul has a different agenda to that of the conscious ego. It sometimes seems that there is something in us that steers our lives in a direction of its own choosing. It can frustrate our plans and thwart our conscious ego's impassioned intentions to remain in charge of our life's direction. When we have accepted and lived out our una-voidable fate it sometimes then becomes more clear who we really are and what life lessons we have needed to learn in order to become more complete as human beings. What is this unknown something that comes to us and presents us with sometimes painful challenges and dis-eases that are not of our own choosing? What is this something that seems to know us so intimately and makes such insistent demands upon us? Is it blind chance? Is it our deeper authentic self? Is it something with a purpose that originates in some mysterious way from beyond our personal selves?

Once again the Greeks offer us a myth that can potentially lead to an intuitive understanding. In *The Myth of Er* Plato offers us an account of the life of the soul between its incarnations in a physical body. Although it is a much briefer and less explicit description of life in the Otherworld it bears some similarities to the better known Bardo Thodol or Tibetan Book of the Dead. The myth was reportedly revealed in a near death and out of body experience. The story tells of a brave warrior by the name of Er. Er was to all appearances killed in battle. His body however remained sound and did not decompose as did those of his other fallen comrades. Nevertheless after twelve days he was put upon a funeral pyre. There he came back to life and was able to speak of his experience of the life of the soul between incarnations. He said that he had been instructed by the beings in the between-world to deliver an account of his experiences for the benefit of the living.

He spoke of the journey of the soul from the body, of its confronta-tion with the "Judges" of the Otherworld, of rewards and punishments, and of the eventual process of reincarnation. In this story we gain an intuitive insight into the nature of the relationship between the con-scious mind and soul.

The disincarnate soul was brought into contact for a number of days with the souls of others who were recently deceased. Together this assembly eventually faced an overwhelming vision of the "spindle of Necessity" from which the tapestry of life itself is woven. This tapestry gives rise to cosmic designs and patterns of which we as individuals are but tiny threads. The goddess "Necessity" (Ananke) was regarded by the Greeks as the primal power in the universe. This goddess was considered to be beyond comprehension or the power of any mortal to control. The gods themselves were subject to her. What must be must be. Here the soul encountered the three Fates or "daughters of Necessity". They were called Lachesis, Clotho, and Atropos. Lachesis was said to "sing" of things past, Clotho of the present, and Atropos of things to come. Sometimes this is depicted as she who spins the thread, she who weaves, and she who cuts it when the pattern is complete.

It was Lachesis who proclaimed to the souls that another round of earthly life was to begin. She cast before them a number of lots which determined the order in which they were allowed to choose their own new incarnation. A number of lives "of every conceivable kind" (Plato, 1955, p. 398) were then spread before them on the ground. This number was said to be "far more" than the number of souls who were invited to choose. In the order of their lot, they were then asked to choose a life that they wished to live.

Each soul freely chose a life based upon its values and aspirations, its wisdom, or its folly and was thus responsible for its choice. The myth makes it clear that the character that one brings to ones chosen life, the sense one makes of ones circumstances, and the values that we hold are not predetermined. They are the responsibilities of the soul. After this choice the soul was bound by Necessity to fulfil its destiny and to live the life of its own choosing.

In order to remind it of its life choice each soul was then invited to choose a "personal daimon" (or what in Christian terminology is sometimes referred to as a "guardian angel") to guide it through its life in order to fulfil its choice. Such a guide was necessary because the souls were then led to the River Lethe or River of Forgetfulness where they were compelled to drink from its waters. Wise souls drank sparingly and were thus able to retain some sense of this between-world with its trials, demands, and commitments.

So, in this myth we are told that our life is of our own choosing even though we have of necessity forgotten our choice. A well-known Jungian analyst once gave a lecture in which he spoke of a luminous dream he once had. In this dream he was able to see with great clarity the whole of his life's plan. In spite of the dream's clarity and power and despite his passionate interest in dreams it evaporated before he could commit it to memory. Although frustrated, he felt in retrospect that to hold such knowledge in consciousness would have undermined his ability to learn and to cope with his circumstances. To know our fate and destiny with certainty would sabotage our ability to learn life's lessons and meet its challenges. Hence in the myth we find the necessity to drink from the waters of forgetfulness.

To compensate for this necessary forgetfulness the myth has it that we are each endowed with a personal daimon or "guardian angel" of our own choice. "Daimon" is a Greek word that refers to a lesser god or spirit. In its original meaning it referred specifically such a spirit who distributed or allotted destinies. The philosopher Socrates wrote of the guidance he received from his daimon. It came to him as a sort of voice that would tell him when *not* to act upon his intentions. The poet W. B. Yeats wrote that he thought of his life as a "struggle with the daimon" (1959, p. 356) who, he felt, set him the hardest tasks that were yet possible for him to do. We have seen too how Jung's personal daimon Philemon introduced him to the idea of the "objective psyche".

We learn from the myth that each of us has an intimate connection with a daimon that can assist us in finding meaning and purpose in our lives. We may ask such philosophical and spiritual questions as— What is the purpose of my life? What is the bigger pattern of which I am a part? What have I come here to do and to learn? We are told that something within us or connected to us is tasked with the job of reminding us of that which we unconsciously already know and are thus capable of recognising and remembering. The answer to our questions comes from an unconscious forgotten aspect of the soul that is connected via the daimon to processes that extend far beyond our personal concerns.

The task of the daimon is to remind us. The daimon is that power within us that enables us to connect with our deeper truth. The task of the soul is to listen. There are those exceptional souls like Socrates and Jung who spontaneously have direct and convincing experiences of such guidance coming to them. But the myth insists that this is a universal human experience. How can the psychotherapist who is an attendant of the soul recognise, understand, and facilitate the dynamic to which the myth refers and thus enable the client or patient to find meaning and purpose? If we are able to do this we might at the least help to achieve Freud's aim of turning neurotic misery into ordinary unhappiness. More than that however, we can aim to facilitate the process of reconnection to meaning, to our life's purpose, and to energies that go beyond the individual. We do this via the daimon or interface between this world and the world beyond. In this way we help to reconnect with the greater planetary and historic tapestry of which the individual person is but a thread. Such a reconnection may invigorate and heal both psychologically and physically.

Growing down

The psychologist James Hillman offered us an alternative way to view psychological processes that takes account of the personal daimon. Psychodynamic and psychoanalytic psychotherapy take a developmental view of the psyche. We imagine that we "grow up" psychologically. We suppose that we become the person that we are today as a result of our life's learning and experience. We look to early experiences to try to reach the source of psychological issues that we face as adults. For example our difficulties in forming intimate relationships in the present day may be thought to have their origins in our early developmental issues with the primary care giver.

Some therapies such as primal therapy and holotropic breath work look even earlier. They look to the birth process itself and even to life in the womb in order to account for the formation of our adult personalities. Useful and insightful though these approaches inarguably are, they contain an assumption that the personality is built from the ground up, that what we are is inherently dependent on our early experiences and learning.

But what if we considered an alternative possibility? Namely that we arrive in the world as complete people; with a character and a life task that we are here to fulfil. We then do not see to be the case that our lives are moulded by our experience, so much as it is that our experiences enable us to become the people that we already are. Hillman calls this the "acorn theory". We are complete in ourselves from the start. An acorn is destined to become an oak and nothing else, whatever the environmental conditions that it encounters. Similarly each of us has a character and a calling. Early experience may help or hinder the process of self manifestation but the goal of a successfully lived life is predetermined.

He offers the story of the film director Martin Scorsese's early years as an example of how we might take this different view with regard to illness. He says of him that he was:

> [...] a very short kid and had terrible asthma. He couldn't go out into the streets of Little Italy in Manhattan and play with the other kids. So he would sit up in his room and look out the window at what was going on and make little drawings—cartoons, with numerous frames—of the scene. In effect he was making movies at nine years old. (Safransky et al., 2012)

In this case we consider the possibility that the illness was in the service of the daimon. It served the purpose of enabling a predestined talent to emerge. In this case the illness seems to have facilitated Scorsese's potential more than it blocked it. When we speak of a "personal daimon" we are referring to this inbuilt sense of our true character and calling, our destiny. Like the oak we not only grow up as we develop, we also grow down. We deepen our roots into the earth as we manifest in earthly form the person who we are predetermined to be.

The royal road

How do we hear the voice of the personal daimon? Freud said that "the interpretation of dreams is the royal road to a knowledge of the unconscious activities of the mind" (1900a). He meant that because dreams are a spontaneous creative activity they give a deep insight into the workings of the unconscious mind.

There is of course an exception to Freud's observation in the widely researched phenomenon of the "lucid dream" in which the dreamer is able to retain a degree of conscious awareness while in "rapid eye movement" (REM) sleep. In this lucid state the dreamer can exercise a degree of autonomy, choice, and control over how the images unfold and develop. In some Buddhist traditions this skill has been highly refined and developed. Nevertheless, for most of us the dream is an experience which is largely beyond the control of the ego. Indeed the ego can often appear as a character in the dream indicating that the psyche is coming from a very different perspective to that with which we are familiar in our waking lives.

This royal road is potentially available to us all. When we experience the contents of the psyche from a perspective other than that of the waking ego we are open to subtle and unfamiliar energies that might otherwise be ignored or suppressed as we arrange our experiences into forms and concepts that are familiar and understandable to ourselves and to the culture of which we are a part. If something new is to enter the psyche, something which we have not already felt, thought, or perceived in consciousness then the dream does indeed provide a "road" or means of access.

Some believe that this ability to perceive the contents of the psyche extends our awareness beyond the "id" or "it" of Freud's imagining. The contents of the psyche can be understood to be more than the images of primal instinctual urges or repressed impulses. They can also be considered to include images of archetypal forces that feed into us as individuals from processes that happen on familial, social, biological, and even cosmic levels. To this extent we may be able to contemplate a connection to forces beyond our individual selves. If we are able to consider how these forces relate to us personally, then to this extent we are talking about something akin to what the Greeks called the personal daimon.

When we look at the inner life in this way we are not talking of "only the imagination" or "just the imagination" as though the imagination were a by-product of our conscious rational self. We are instead regarding the imagination as a mode of perception, a way of encountering energies and phenomena that are present to us but otherwise beyond the power of our physical senses to perceive. We have noted how the philosopher and theologian Henry Corbin uses the word "imaginal" to make a distinction between the imagination as a mode of perception from the dismissive and belittling colloquial use of the word.

However, with regard to the voice of the daimon, the royal road is not the only road. Although sleep laboratories have demonstrated that everyone dreams, not everyone is easily able to recall their dreams. In psychotherapy some psychotherapists employ any of a variety of techniques such as active imagination or guided fantasy in order to tune into the images of the unconscious mind. These methods aim to create a trancelike state in which images spontaneously present themselves to consciousness and may then be worked with in the way we might work with a dream. We hope to reveal significance and meaning. If we approach things this way the psychotherapist or client has to some extent already predetermined what to look for. The values and choices of the conscious ego begin to colour the nature of what will be revealed.

Robert Sardello explains it this way:

> Creating activity is strongest with the dream, for there it is most free. This element is still present in fantasy, although more bound to the ego—the ego is always at the centre of our fantasy life, with imaginary pictures serving the wishes of the ego. With memory a creating element is still present, but is now bound to an event that occurred in the outer world. Thus memory recalls events that have happened, but does not do this in a completely literal way. With thinking, the creating element is bound to the laws of logic, which brings an orderly relation between one thought and another. When this orderly element is lacking, we have something approaching free association rather than thinking. And, with perception, the creating element is most bound by what is actually present before us. Nonetheless, even in perception there is an aspect of creating what we see, as evidenced by the possibility of illusion. (1995, p. 112)

We have here a graded scale beginning with the most subtle and intuitive powers of the imagination and ending in the most concrete. We go from dream, to fantasy, to memory, to thought, and to perception. We can see that although the imagination is a necessary part of all of our experience, we lose our capacity to appreciate its "otherness" as we work our way from an openness to the dream to a literalist attitude of "seeing is believing" at the level of perception. Earlier we saw how Dethlefsen and Dahlke offered us a similar scale by which we could see how psychological issues that are not encountered or resolved on a psychological level become progressively more deeply imbedded in the physical body. If we cannot hear the message of the dream or the voice of the daimon in the dream we may find it necessary to respond to a more compelling manifestation of the image. We may struggle with physical circumstances that come to us either in the outer world or from the inner world in terms of psychological or physical symptoms and illness.

If there are psychobiological issues that require our attention, they grow ever more insistent as we move along the scale from the intuitive perception of them to the fully manifest dis-ease. Referring to this subtle level of imaginal perceptions as "premonitions" archetypal psychologist Alfred Ziegler says that:

> [...] premonitions are always present, in one way or another [...]. Pre-morbid premonitions support health, precede disease,

and guide those of us who pay attention on the path of physical well-being. (1983, p. 12)

If we listen to the whisper of the dream and make the necessary changes we may not need to hear the shouts of the fully manifest dis-ease.

The daimon

We have noted that the word daimon originally referred to an entity that delivered ones destiny by linking life in this world to a world beyond; a world where ones life's purpose was predetermined. The daimon was regarded as a lesser god or spirit who served as an intermediary between the worlds. It was believed to partake of the nature of both worlds and to be confined to neither. At a time long before the Cartesian divide of the seventeenth century, it was considered to be a paradoxical being. Because it belonged to both worlds it could not be said to be a strictly spiritual being nor could it be accurately described as a physical one. The Christian church shared this view and recognised the existence of the daimon. They referred to it as the "Guardian Angel". The existence of such an entity became part of Christian dogma at the Council of Nicaea in the year 325. However, over five centuries later at the Church Council of 869 in Constantinople it was established in dogma that man was composed of two parts only; namely body and spirit. The psyche (or soul) and the daimon were then regarded as aspects of the spiritual side of life which required the guidance of the priests of the church. What had been regarded as the intermediate realm of the psyche and its daimon was then deprived of its ambivalent, paradoxical and earthly nature.

The physical environment and the body became disconnected from the psyche or soul which until that time had embraced both the worlds of spirit and that of matter. We learned to deal with events in the physical realm as though they bore no direct relationship to our destiny or life's purpose. The church had failed to heed the warning of the Greek philosopher Plutarch who lived in Rome at the very beginning of the Christian era. He said that those who deny the existence of the daimons "make the relations of gods and men remote and alien [...] and force us to a disorderly confusion in things" (1936, p. 389). We could begin to imagine the possibility of a purely spiritual realm that had no connection to our physicality.

We can see that the daimon straddled both worlds and belonged to neither. The Anglo-Irish philosophical writer Patrick Harpur describes the daimonic realm in this way:

> Never quite divine nor quite human, the daimons erupted out of the Soul of the World. They were neither spiritual nor physical, but both. Neither were they, as Jung discovered wholly inner nor wholly outer, but both. They were paradoxical beings, both good and bad, benign and frightening, guiding and warning, protecting and maddening. (1994, pp. 37–38)

Existential psychotherapist Rollo May elaborates on the paradoxical and ambivalent nature of the daimon by saying that "the daimonic refers to the power of nature rather than to the superego, and is beyond good and evil" (1969, p. 124). Being a natural phenomenon it cannot be said to be good or evil any more than could any other natural force such as the wind, rain, fire, or earth. Hurricanes, floods, forest fires and earthquakes, like the daimons, are natural phenomena beyond moral or ethical evaluation.

However, as Christianity increasingly became the dominant context in which to try to understand the nature of psyche or soul, the term daimon lost its ambivalent and paradoxical nature. The Guardian Angel was considered to be aligned wholly with the good angelic realms. The term daimon came to be replaced by the word "demon" which usually refers to a malevolent spirit. It was believed that entities that were not aligned with the Christian faith could only be regarded as misleading and hindrances to the possibility of salvation. They were therefore negative and in needed to be avoided. The daimons thus became not only split off from the material world but also came to be regarded as "demonic".

Psychotherapy is concerned with pathology. The business of psychotherapy is to attend to those disruptive and disturbing symptoms that bring clients into therapy. It is the pain and disturbance of what goes wrong in life that engenders the urge and impulse to attend psychotherapy. There the process of working with the troubling symptoms, the illnesses, the dis-eases of both body and soul can lead to deep reflection, learning, expanded consciousness, and re-evaluation of life. Sometimes the presenting pathologies will ease or resolve as the underlying issues are addressed with greater consciousness and deeper reflection. Sometimes it may be possible to live with greater acceptance and equanimity with conditions that persist.

Those physical and psychological troubles from which clients long to be freed and with which conventional medicine is prepared to wage war can contain within them the possibility of a fuller degree of awareness and health in the sense of wholeness. Like the personal daimon illness is paradoxical. It is not a good thing to be ill. Nor ultimately is it a bad thing to be ill. It is both good and bad to be ill. It is neither good nor bad to be ill. It is a paradoxical natural force, an inevitable inescapable aspect of being an incarnate human being. It cannot be evaluated in terms of moral worth. Illness is daimonic.

The paradox of illllness

There is an old Chinese story that illustrates well the moral ambiguity of apparent misfortune. It concerns the fortunes of a kindly impoverished farmer who was brought the news that his loving father (who lived in a distant province) had died. His neighbours came to console him in his misfortune but he could not agree that he had indeed suffered a misfortune.

Some while later his relatives brought to him a fine and valuable horse that had been left to him by his father. His neighbours wanted to celebrate their delight in his good fortune but again he could not agree that he had been fortunate.

When the horse wandered off and became lost the neighbours again wished to console him in his bad luck. And again he could not agree that this was necessarily bad. The next day he found his horse together with another wild horse and was able to bring them both back to his farm. There the neighbours of course congratulated him on his apparent good fortune. Later however his son tried to tame the wild horse but was thrown from it and broke his leg making him unable to help with the harvest. But perhaps it was not the bad fortune it appeared to be because the very next day the king's army arrived. They were there to draft new recruits to fight in a war. His son had the apparent good fortune to be spared.

If we are able to look deeply and patiently enough at the seeming adversity and misfortune of illness we may begin to see it differently. This has certainly been the experience of a number of writers who have written movingly and eloquently about their encounters with illness.

Jill Bolte-Taylor was a medical researcher when she suffered a severe incapacitating stroke while on her own at home. She says it "stripped my mind of its ability to recall the memories and details of my previous life", leaving her "like an infant" (2008, p. 65). She is able to say in retrospect:

> What a wonderful gift this stroke has been in permitting me to pick and choose who and how I want to be in the world. Before the stroke I believed I was a product of this brain and that I had minimal say about how I felt or what I thought. Since the haemorrhage, my eyes have been opened to how much choice I actually have about what goes on between my ears. (2008, p. 122)

Similarly the writer Kat Duff is able to say of her long encounter with chronic fatigue and immune dysfunction syndrome (CFIDS):

> [...] it seems clear to me that one of the tasks of illness, and requirements of healing, is to reclaim ones soul—that vital essence that enables us to thrive—and resume ones "path of destiny". (1993, p. 74)

Albert Kreinheder was a Jungian analyst who wrote thoughtfully and movingly of his experience of aging and his impending death with terminal illnesses. He was aware of having an inner spirit guide or daimon who instructed him thus:

> The paradox is that the wound, the illness, is also the treasure. The physical misery gets your attention. But then if you go deeper, there is much more to it, memories and imagination and worries of what will come [...]. That's where the treasure is, in the psychic images that come with the symptoms. The symptoms open you up. They literally tear you open so the things you need can flow in. (1991, pp. 53–54)

An extreme example of this experience of being "torn open" is described vividly by Sandra Lee Dennis who suffered a frightening predominantly psychological "breakdown" or perhaps we should say "breakthrough".

> Horrifying demonic figures broke into my mind at odd hours of the day and night. Vivid sado-masochistic scenes erupted from

nowhere, along with dismemberment, scatology, rape, incest, and a sense of satanic possession. My inner life teemed with strange images of ax-murderers, rapists, tarantulas, rats, maggots, snakes. I was deeply disturbed by the insistent reality of these awful images. (2001, p. 2)

She describes how she was able to work psychologically with repeated bouts of this kind of lurid imagery and the physical bodily sensations that accompanied it. These intrusions into her conscious mind occurred over a period of years. She regarded them as challenge proffered to her by the daimonic realms and as a necessary part of her life's work.

The daimon can dement or enlighten, sicken or vitalize, destroy or nurture. If we, in the depths of the subtle body, accept and embrace its energy pattern, the unique presence of the daimon, it releases its "redeeming" aspects—the essential wisdom, or strength, or beauty, for example, at the heart of the image. (2001, p. 119)

We can see from the work of these writers that there is a potentially liberating power to be found within our symptoms and illnesses. This is the case whether they are at the very subtle level of the dream or at the all too tangible and compelling levels of physical illness and even of death. The daimon continues to speak in the world today. Those who have the ears to hear and the conceptual frameworks within which to begin to understand it can best profit from its messages. To facilitate and to support this process, in other words to "attend to soul", is the job of psychotherapy.

CHAPTER SEVEN

The daimonic bodymind

To see a World in a Grain of Sand
And a Heaven in a Wild Flower,
Hold Infinity in the palm of your hand
And Eternity in an hour.

—*William Blake* (1946, p. 150)

et us try to get a sense of the nature of the daimonic by considering the ways in which we regard time. There are three terms we normally employ in regard to the passage of time; namely we consider that events occur in the past, the present, and the future. When we look more closely however it is ever more difficult to locate an event that actually occurs in the present. It is possible to measure time in terms of nanoseconds or billionth parts of seconds. Researchers say that in the body "depending on the type of fiber, the neural impulse travels at speeds ranging from a sluggish 2 miles per hour to, in some myelinated fibers, a breakneck 200 or more miles per hour. But even this top speed is 3 million times slower than the speed of electricity through a wire" (Myers, 1986, p. 43). We can see that nerve impulses take time to reach their destinations. By the time we are aware that our hand has reflexively withdrawn itself from a red hot object the event is already in the past. The to-ing and fro-ing of nerve impulses has taken time. If we think of time in this way it is as though the past is a vast scarcely imaginable span stretching back to the origins of the universe. Similarly the future stretches out before us in an unimaginable way. When we think in this way we might well ask if the present moment exists at all. Perhaps the present moment is only a construct or hypothesis. It is the thinnest of thin lines that divides the two awe inspiring immeasurable mysteries of past and future. We know that when we gaze at the stars, the objects we see are as they were in the depths of the past. So too when we look closely we find that even apparently immediate sensory experiences do in fact require time to be conveyed to our awareness.

However we can reverse this way of thinking. We can understand time in the more immediate, sensual, embodied, and soulful way that Blake does in his poem. We can consider the irrefutable fact that there is only the present moment. Experientially speaking nothing has ever happened or will ever happen in any moment other than the present. It is all we have. It is all we have ever had, and all we ever will have. We have only the present moment. When we look at our experience in this way the past and future become insubstantial hypothetical constructs that have no sensory reality. They are merely mental constructs that serve as sometimes useful tools that help us to navigate our way through the eternal present in which we live our lives.

American philosopher David Abram says that he has a way of restoring this sense of soulful embodiment when he feels he's fallen into what he calls the "civilised oblivion of linear time."

> I locate myself in a relatively open space—a low hill is particularly good, or a wide field. I relax a bit, take a few breaths, gaze around. Then I let myself begin to feel the whole bulk of my past—the whole mass of events leading up to this very moment. And I call into awareness, as well, my whole future—all those projects and possibilities that lie waiting to be realized. I imagine this past and this future as two vast balloons of time, separated from each other like the bulbs of an hourglass, yet linked together at the moment when I stand pondering them. And then, very slowly, I allow both these immense globes of time to begin leaking their substance into this minute moment between them, into the present.

Slowly, imperceptibly at first, the present moment begins to grow. Nourished by the leakage from the past and the future, the present moment swells in proportion as those other elements shrink. Soon it is very large; and the past and future have dwindled down to mere knots at the end of this huge expanse. At this point I let the past and the future dissolve entirely. And I open my eyes [...]. (1996, p. 202)

If we can grasp a sense of that to which William Blake and David Abram refer we can also sense something of the nature of the daimonic, the soul, or the psyche. From the point of view of dualistic Cartesian thinking this soul realm is a mere nothing. Yet from within its own perspective it is reality itself. It joins and encompasses both the material and spiritual realms. It brings life and significance to the material realm while it grounds abstract spirituality in the sensual.

We have seen that when we look at the task of psychotherapy from this daimonic perspective we become interested in the impact and significance of illness and its symptoms. We make less of a divide between conditions that manifest in a predominantly invisible emotional way such as anxiety and depression and those that are more tangible and evidently physical. We have seen that many writers and sufferers are able to see meaning and purpose in the most extreme and overwhelming of physical afflictions.

Susan Sontag

On the other hand there are those such as the influential American writer and filmmaker Susan Sontag who took exception and offence at the idea that her life threatening cancer might be regarded as anything other than a strictly physical condition. She felt that:

[...] the metaphorical trappings that deform the experience of having cancer have very real consequences: they inhibit people from seeking treatment early enough, or from making greater effort to get competent treatment. The metaphors and myths, I was convinced, kill (For instance, they make people irrationally fearful of effective measures such as chemotherapy, and foster credence in thoroughly useless remedies such as diets and psychotherapy). (1989, pp. 99–100)

"Metaphors kill" she declares. And yes maybe sometimes they do. This is especially so if they are taken literally as an alternative to treatment. The job of the daimon, the soul, and of psychotherapy is to occupy the space between the split polarities of gross, literal physicality and an invisible, disembodied, transcendent spirituality. The daimon holds the worlds together. "Metaphor" is a term that we can use to understand how it does this. Metaphor means to "carry beyond" (Greek; *meta* equals beyond, *pherein* equals to carry). In modern Greek the word "metaphor" is used to denote a mode of transportation. In Greece one can quite "literally" climb aboard a "metaphor" to get from one geographical place to another. In psychotherapy we aim to assist in the process of healing by retaining sensitivity and openness to the greater forces at work even if this be in a time of crisis. We aim to assist a sufferer in the natural daimonic process of being "carried beyond" the place of literal and seemingly meaningless physical or mental suffering to a place wherein they can find significance. The daimonic perspective takes nothing away from physically orientated medical intervention. Instead it connects it to the dimension of meaning and purpose.

Sontag insists that an acute physical disease must be dealt with immediately in a practical physical way. It has no "meaning" and occurs by chance. For her, as for many people today, disease does not raise anything more than physical and practical implications. The realms of matter and spirit remain distinct and divorced from one another without the connecting principle of psyche, soul, and daimon with its language of symbols and metaphors. She stresses that disease is "not a curse, not a punishment, not an embarrassment." She felt that cancer had been stigmatised with just these attributes at the time she first suffered from the condition in the 1970s. We are reminded of the story of Job in the Biblical Old Testament. His friends, in their avowed intention of helping and comforting him, instead insisted that his suffering must be a kind of punishment from God for his terrible sins despite his having lived a faultless and spiritually devoted life. Thus they added to his struggle by withholding compassion and attributing personal blame to him for his suffering.

We can agree with Susan Sontag when she rightly points out that personal blame is not helpful to someone burdened by disease and even less helpful when someone is frightened for their survival. We can agree too that we as sufferers are most certainly *not* responsible *for* our accidents, symptoms, and illnesses. Nor is metaphor helpful as a way of drawing our attention to our inadequacies, insufficiencies, and failures in life. Some New Agers may disagree but we *can* in fact afford the luxury of a negative thought. We don't need to walk on the sunny side of the street. In order to be real we can and must have the experience we are having. Psychotherapy does not blame and burden the sufferer. Nor does it suggest that they are responsible for their condition.

However we do suggest that a client can be responsible *to* the condition. That is to say that it is possible to be "able to respond" creatively to even the most adverse of conditions. By allowing the connection to what is unconsciously emerging to be realised we aim to facilitate the process of becoming more whole; in other words the process of "healing". To do this we work in cooperation with the daimonic energy contained within the symptom. To imagine oneself responsible for a condition is to take ownership of it. It suggests that the ego is in charge. To respond to a condition by contrast indicates humility and openness. We are presented with something autonomous that requires our response. When we relate to our pathology through the imagination in this way we allow its daimonic energy to "flow in" to us or "influence" us. This energy lessens our egocentricity while it increases our potential, enlarges our consciousness, and makes us more whole.

Richard

Let us consider the place of the daimon in relation to cancer by considering the case of Richard. Richard was a highly educated and successful man in his sixties who had made a name for himself as an architect and also as university lecturer. Until ten years before coming to psychotherapy he had been passionately involved in and committed to his creative work. He was so fervently absorbed that he often worked late into the night on projects. His enthusiasm was such that he said he felt himself at times to be almost "possessed". He had had numerous relationships with women before he met his present partner about twenty years ago. After ten years together he married this partner, and shortly after this he was diagnosed with prostate cancer. Following the diagnosis he said that he felt his "life was no longer his own". His energy levels dropped and he was obliged to deal with the medical complications and challenges that were to follow. He was treated both with radiotherapy and with "brachytherapy". This involved implanting tiny radioactive "seeds" or wires into the prostate in order to kill the cancer. He was fortunate insofar as the cancer was contained within the prostate, so it was possible to avoid its removal and further potential consequences such as impotency and urinary incontinence which might have followed from this.

He was additionally given hormone therapy. In the case of prostate cancer sufferers, this typically requires large amounts of the "female" hormone estrogen. By contrast in cases of cervical cancers large amounts of the "male" hormone testosterone are sometimes given as a treatment. For Richard this resulted in breast swelling which for cosmetic reasons needed to be dealt with surgically.

These health problems made it necessary for him to retire early even though in his words his "work was his life". With the intention of reducing his stress levels he and his wife eventually felt it was wise to move away from the busy and stressful urban environments that had supported his career. They opted instead to live near the sea in a quiet town in a remote but beautiful part of the country.

As the illness progressively came under control Richard's energy gradually returned. In part his recovered energy expressed itself after a couple of drinks in angry frustrated temper outbursts and a growing intolerance of the sleepy parochial small town ways of the place in which he lived. This was brought to his attention by his wife who felt disturbed and intimidated by his sudden flares of anger. Although Richard was a big assertive man with a deep voice and a commanding presence, he found it hard to understand how his wife could feel disturbed by his outbursts which seemed to him entirely proportionate and appropriate to the frustrating situations with which he dealt.

On the contrary, Richard felt that he was self-reliant and self-contained. He prided himself on his inner creative resources. He believed that he was perfectly happy to pursue his creative interests on his own at home with his main social and professional contacts being made over the internet. The issue that brought him to psychotherapy was that he didn't know how to manage with his wife. In his view she was becoming increasingly intolerant and unreasonable in her demands of him. She had become uncertain that she wished to continue the relationship. She insisted that he involve himself more in the local community and curb what was in his view an honest outspokenness on which he prided himself. She felt that he "needed to do some work on himself" if he wanted to save the marriage.

Until his marriage and diagnosis Richard's "work was his life". After these two events his "life was no longer his own". He transformed from a highly energised and motivated man whose main preoccupation and fulfilment in life was his creative work, to a man who had suddenly become dependent and vulnerable. He needed the support of medical professionals to keep him alive and the support of his wife in order to deal with the physical and emotional trials he was experiencing. His was a sudden transition from what some might call a "human doing" to a human being. He was forced to become more aware of his body, his vulnerability, and his need for emotional and physical support from others.

His cancer of the prostate, that exclusively male organ, and its uncontrolled growth put the future survival of the whole of his organism under threat. The disease threatened death and demanded a kind of rebirth. The life with which he had been identified came to an abrupt end even as his new life as a married man and a medical patient began. Medically and literally speaking one of the things that was required to restore his health or wholeness was a large dose of the "female" hormone estrogen. He was given a dose large enough that he actually began to embody some physical aspects of the feminine. Psychologically we can ask whether a parallel process was occurring. Perhaps he needed to develop some "feminine" psychological characteristics. The illness obliged him to open up in his life by becoming more aware of his body, his vulnerability, and his emotionality—qualities that in our culture tend to be better developed in women than in men. These parallel processes can be thought of as daimonic in that they join and unite the invisible and visible dimensions of health. Jung says that:

> The distinction between mind and body is an artificial dichotomy, an act of discrimination based far more on the peculiarity of intellectual cognition than on the nature of things. (1921, p. 254)

The illness is simultaneously both a literal physical illness and a psychological state. In this case the metaphor of masculine and feminine qualities is useful if and only if it can "carry us beyond" the literal. If a metaphor leads to self-discovery and self-realisation we know we are working psychotherapeutically. Metaphor can be a potent agent of healing or wholing.

Richard's dream life revealed something of the nature of the changes that he went through during the course of the twenty months of his psychotherapy. His initial dreams were virtually all retrospective. They took him back to the times, places, and people of his past. People and places were jumbled together associating disparate events and prompting reflection on hidden patterns in his life that had brought him to the present crisis in his identity and in his relationship.

The dreams became increasingly vivid and compelling. They came to something of a climax around half way through his therapy when he dreamed that he was presented with a diploma by the Architectural Registration Board. The vivid and unforgettable thing about this image was the fact that he found that he had got out of bed in his sleep. He woke to find himself standing in the middle of his bedroom with his arm outstretched ready to receive his diploma. The dream impressed him with the fact that he needed recognition and validation from the outside world. It became evident that he was not quite the independent and emotionally self-sufficient person he liked to think that he was. As Jung says:

> The daimon throws us down, makes us traitors to our ideals and cherished convictions—traitors to the selves we thought we were. (1956, p. 357)

The angry outbursts at the frustrations of small town life were indicative that his returning energy required a new sense of self and new creative outlets.

He found that he was able to do exactly this over the second half of his psychotherapeutic work. He found ways of working part time in the city while at the same time involving himself in the local community. He found more value in the insights offered to him by his wife and indeed by the "feminine" qualities within himself. By the end of his therapy his dreams were of "new road layouts", "going 'on the road'" and "packing his car with his suitcase and his dog ready to go".

Illness as a metaphor

> Man has no Body distinct from his Soul; for that call'd Body is a portion of Soul discern'd by the five Senses, the chief inlets of Soul in this age. (1946, p. 250)

> William Blake

When we ask "what is it like" to have a particular symptom or condition we enter into metaphorical thinking. From head to foot every part and function of the body is psychological as well as literal and physical. The metaphor bridges the gap between. A headache for example is literally an ache in the head. At the same time it is an annoying and persistent problem that confounds a clear resolution. A sore foot may indicate that we are taking a painful step.

When we become sensitive to the language of metaphor we enter the realm of the daimonic; or that principle which unites tangible physical reality with the invisible psychological and spiritual dimensions of life. Freud described the dream as the Royal Road to the unconscious. That same road is also to be found in our symptoms and our illnesses. Only in this case we are obliged to take note. We cannot simply turn over and forget as we might forget a dream. Depending on the gravity of the symptom or illness we must use a full range of resources in order to address that which confronts us. Freud's mentor in psychosomatic medicine was the physician Georg Groddeck. Writing in the 1930s Groddeck emphasised his practical priorities when he stressed that if he were to treat a patient with an open wound, that "the bleeding must be stopped first before any other measures can be thought of" (1970, p. 194). However when we have addressed the most tangible and literal aspects of a condition with conventional medicine we are in a position to begin the healing task of actual psychotherapy or psychotherapy that "actually" does justice to its task of attending to the needs of the soul. In this case we must disagree with Susan Sontag; the metaphor does not kill but heals.

In Groddeck's view there is a "force" within us that has some kind of intent or end in mind for us. What he describes is reminiscent of what we have been calling the personal daimon. He says that because the force carries out such "marvellous processes" as fashioning the whole of our physical bodies he therefore does not:

> [...] find it unreasonable to suppose that it can even manufacture pneumonia or gout or cancer. I dare go so far with my patients as to maintain that the force really does such things, that according to its pleasure it makes people ill for specific ends, that according to its pleasure it selects for such ends the place, the time and the nature of the illness. (1923, p. 100)

What ends might "the force" or the daimon intend? How can psychotherapy attend to this process? How can we hear and interpret the language of illness and its symptoms so that we can serve the needs of the soul?

Frederick Perls, the founder of gestalt psychotherapy, was another early writer on the subject of how the body expresses psychological processes. In the 1940s he made his view clear that he, like Jung, and Blake, felt that there was no true division between body and soul. He said that "the words 'body' and 'soul' denote two aspects of the same thing", and "No emotion [...] occurs without its physiological as well as psychological components coming into play" (1947, pp. 33–34). If we accept this premise we may conclude that physiological phenomena without accompanying emotions invite exploration in search of unconscious emotions.

In his revision of psychoanalysis he draws many illuminating parallels between psychological and physiological processes. He finds equivalences between the way the body processes food and the mind processes experience or "mental food". Both experience and food need to be taken into the bodymind if we are to gain nourishment from them. He gives a number of very clear examples as to how psychological issues in this regard can become manifest in very real biological and medical conditions.

Take the case of a patient who suffers from a gastric or duodenal ulcer for example. A bleeding sore in the stomach lining is a painful and unequivocal physical condition. It is not imaginary in the sense of being "made up" in order to obtain secondary gains such as sympathy or to avoid certain situations though both of these may follow as a result of the condition.

The stomach is inarguably a vital physical organ of the body. If we agree that body and mind are two aspects of the same thing it is equally indisputable that the stomach is a psychological phenomenon. Metaphor, soul, or the daimonic is the bridge that links and unites these two aspects of the whole. We get a sense of what we might begin to consider with such a stomach complaint in everyday metaphorical language. What is it that we can't "stomach" or digest? What are we hungry for? What can we not swallow? Have we swallowed so much that we are "fed up" and "cannot take any more"? and so on. We intuitively recognise the parallel between food and mental food. Perls reminds us:

> [...] that the stomach is just a kind of skin, unable to deal with lumps. Sometimes the organism, in order to compensate for the

> lack of chewing, produces an excessive quantity of stomach acid
> and pepsin. This adjustment, however, entails the development of
> a gastric or duodenal ulcer. (1947, p. 109)

But then why would a person not chew their food either physically or
psychologically? Firstly there are cultural factors. It is true that we live
in a fast food culture and an "information society" wherein we can be
overloaded with images and ideas. Collective forces make it easy for us
to swallow more than we can digest. But why would a person have a
tendency to "swallow things whole" be it food or ideas? Both need to be
chewed over in order to make them digestible so that they may release
their nutrients in order that they might sustain body and mind. The
bodymind is signalling that this behaviour needs to stop. Perhaps mild
indigestion has not done the trick. Soothing and suppressive medications may have kept more subtle symptoms at bay for some considerable time. The whispers may have been overlooked until the condition
shouts loudly enough for it to be heard.

Perls points out that there is a stage in life when it is perfectly healthy
and appropriate to swallow things whole; namely the "oral" stage of
the suckling infant. The question then arises as to what might cause
an adult to eat in a way that imitates this phase of development. Why
would someone eat solid foods as though they were liquid and thus
overburden the stomach. What is the story behind what he calls the
"dental inhibition"? Why the reluctance to be "incisive" to "get ones
teeth into" a source of nourishment, to "chew it over" being careful
not to "swallow things whole" so that it is easily stomached, assimi-
lated and put to good use by the organism. According to psychoanalytic
theory Perls asks what developmental trauma may have occurred in
relation to the mother. Might she perhaps have withdrawn the breast
which at this early stage the infant would not have differentiated from
her love? Perhaps she might even have smacked the baby for being
"naughty" if it bit, thus leaving a lasting inhibition and laying the foundation for a later inability to "get ones teeth" into a task. Perhaps the
foundations would also be laid for a fear of aggression, of being hurt
or of hurting others. Aggressive impulses might then be projected onto
others out there in the exterior world where they would be encountered
as a disowned aspect of the personality.

In the medical view peptic and duodenal ulcers are believed to be
"caused" by a bacterium known as helicobacter pylori. It is a bacterium

that is also very commonly found in the stomach and guts of persons who experience no symptoms and have no problems in this regard. Standard medical treatment for such ulcers is likely to include taking antibiotics and a course of acid suppressing medication. If the treatment is left at this stage then the job is at best only partly and superficially done. If the physical symptom or voice of the daimon is "successfully" suppressed, the message remains unheard; the person does not take a step toward deeper self-awareness. Healing (or wholing) has been avoided, the split between body and mind has been reinforced, and the "force" within the organism that creates disease will be obliged to send a stronger more insistent message if its intent is to be heard. This idea is not new.

> If you bring forth what is within you, what you bring forth will save you. If you do not bring forth what is within you, what you do not bring forth will destroy you.

Said Jesus in the Gospel of Thomas (Miller, 1994, verse 70). Health involves a degree of ego surrender.

"Process oriented" psychotherapist Arnold Mindell demonstrates this principle well when he describes his work with one of his patients. Following an unsuccessful operation, a man he was seeing was dying a painful, "sad and terrifying" death from stomach cancer. "He was lying in the hospital bed, groaning and moaning in pain", says Mindell. However instead of looking for ways to soothe the patient or help him to bear the pain Mindell suggested that he try to make the pain worse. He cooperated.

> He lay on his back and started to increase the pressure in his stomach. He pushed his stomach out and kept pushing and pressing and exaggerating the pain until he felt as if he were going to explode. Suddenly at the height of his pain he shouted out, "Oh Arny, I just want to explode!" (1985, p. 7)

When he had given vocal release to this sensation it suddenly occurred to him that he had never before fully expressed himself. At the end of this physical work the patient felt a great deal better. Although he had been on the verge of death his condition improved to the point that he became well enough to leave hospital. In his further meetings with

Mindell he learned to "explode" in the presence of another person and to give vent to feelings he had not been able to express in the course of his life. He lived for another "two or three years".

Grace

Less acute was the case of Grace, a thirty-year-old woman with whom I worked. Although she was young, attractive, and had a well-paid creative job she had a great sense of inadequacy. She had recently been able to end a seven year relationship with a man who she felt could never return her love. She had overlooked the fact that he slept around with other women on a regular basis. She felt that someone as undeserving as she was lucky to have a man in her life at all.

She was the only child of her parents and had what she called an "idyllic" childhood in New Zealand. She said that as a child she felt that her father was also her best friend. She came to the UK at the age of eleven following the breakup of her parents' marriage. After the breakup her grieving, embittered, "suicidal" mother forbade any contact with her father. Suddenly she had lost her father, her friends, and her familiar surroundings. Grace felt that her mother demanded she take the place of her Dad by insisting that they slept together. "She hung over me like a cloud of obligation and guilt" said Grace. She presented with a dream.

> I am driving along happily in a car with my Dad. There is a little figure like Robin Hood on the dashboard. He draws a bow and shoots me with an arrow. I wake up in panic.

The dream seemed to emphasise the importance of her relationship to her father which was brought to a sudden and devastating end. She said she felt betrayed and disillusioned by him. When in later life she contacted him she found that he was cold and indifferent to her. The Robin Hood figure is a green man of the woods who reminds us of Pan. He duly delivers a "Panic attack". Something "toxic" has gotten under her skin (*toxon* meaning a bow in Greek, *taxa* meaning arrow in Old Persian) that needs to be expressed.

In the course of her therapy which lasted for about a year this is exactly what she did. She "unpacked" what she called a "suitcase full of pain". This came to a somewhat surprising climax one evening when she was at home alone doing the therapeutic exercise of writing a story about "a girl who was angry at her mother". She was startled when she suddenly realised she could see clearly without her prescription lenses. The shock of this terrified her to the point that she needed to support herself in order to stand upright. She could not figure out whether she was terrified that she could see clearly or could see clearly because she was in touch with her terror. What she had for many years accepted as the unremarkable and purely physical problem of near sightedness revealed itself to also be an embodied metaphor. When at last she saw her emotional problems clearly the tensions that underpinned her myopia were released and the condition spontaneously came to an end.

The body is psychological. The psyche is embodied. Seen this way they are daimonic.

CHAPTER EIGHT

The psychophysical environment

John Sarno

John Sarno is an American medical professor. He is one of a number of medical practitioners who recognise the psychological components of illnesses that are generally regarded by both patient and doctor as physically based. He writes about a group of physical conditions which he terms "tension myositis syndrome" or TMS. "Myositis" simply means a physical alteration of the muscles. These conditions include such predominantly muscular conditions as chronic back, neck, and limb pain as well as other problems such as repetitive-strain injuries, gastrointestinal illnesses, and dermatological conditions.

He proposes that the painful chronic and sometimes incapacitating symptoms that sufferers feel:

> [...] are players in a strategy designed to keep our attention focused on the body so as to prevent dangerous feelings from escaping into consciousness or to avoid confrontation with feelings that are unbearable. (1998, p. 18)

Pharmaceutical and physiologically based treatments are therefore unlikely to be effective in dealing with such conditions. To the extent that these treatments offer relief from pain he considers it to be the case that they merely challenge the unconscious mind to devise other strategies to distract us from the unbearable feelings.

He says he would explain to a patient with this condition that they had:

> [...] a harmless condition that must be treated through the mind not the body. Awareness, insight, knowledge and information were the magic medicines that would cure this disorder—and nothing else could do it. (1998, p. xxi)

The "medicine" that he has in mind in order to raise this awareness and to gain this insight and information, is psychoanalytic psychotherapy.

The role of such psychoanalytic healing is to raise awareness of these unbearable feelings and to offer support as a sufferer learns to deal with what they are trying to avoid by the "strategy" of creating physical pain for themselves. The "strategy" takes place subconsciously when we repress the expression of strong emotions. This creates muscular tension. He cites the potentially dangerous and destructive emotion of rage as the expression a patient is most likely to feel the need to hold back. When this tension and withholding are chronic it results in the production of the painful and distracting symptoms.

He reports that raising consciousness of underlying issues and finding appropriate contextualised emotional release enables his patients to find relief from chronic pain. He says that seventy-six per cent of his patients who follow his treatment report that they are able to live virtually pain free lives. Of those with the specific complaint of herniated discs identified on computerised tomography (CT) scans he says his success rate is eighty-eight per cent. His methods have been scientifically backed up by a peer reviewed study showing a fifty-four per cent reduction in pain for sufferers (Schechter, 2007, pp. 26–35).

Sarno's work follows firmly in the footsteps of his predecessor Goerg Groddeck who in the 1920s wrote that would say to a patient with a cold:

> Why have you a nose? To smell with, he replies. So I say, Your It has given you a cold in order that you shall not smell something or other. Find out what it is you are not to smell. And now and again the patient will actually find out some smell which he wants to

escape, and you need not believe it, but I do—when he has found it, the cold disappears. (1923, p. 100)

Both Sarno and Groddeck draw attention to a paradox. They say that the symptom is produced in order to enable us to avoid a psychological issue. Yet at the same time the symptom clearly draws our attention to the issue. We can see an analogy with the matter of self-harming. The semi consciously administered self-inflicted physical pain and visible wounding both diverts attention from and draws attention to the invisible underlying emotional pain. The ego that avoids emotional pain is only one aspect of the psyche. It is the daimonic drive toward wholeness that demands that we attend to that which we wish to avoid. In this way we more fully self-actualise. Again we are reminded of Jesus's words in the Gospel of Thomas. What we face and bring forth will "save" or heal us. What we try to avoid will "destroy" or damage us. We need to get beyond a limited egocentric view of who and what we are in order to be whole, healthy, and indeed "holy". In this way we can see that the ailments grouped under the heading of TMS can be a means to an end as we move toward greater health.

The idea that psychological issues are manifested in the body in the form of chronic tensions has long been accepted in the field of Reichian bodywork. Repressed memories and spontaneous imagery often arise in the course of bodywork such as deep tissue massage and bioenergetics. As tense muscles are stretched and relaxed we can become suddenly conscious of the emotions that we have been holding within. In addition to emotional discharge an image may emerge that enables a client to suddenly recall a long forgotten incident in childhood that has led to a lifelong pattern of holding back or holding in. When this occurs some practitioners then shift the focus of the work from the body to working with the images or memories as one might in a psychotherapy that was not body orientated.

Dutch Jungian psychoanalyst Robert Bosnak addresses this awareness of the psychological nature of the body from the other direction with a method that he calls "embodied imagination". He describes a way of working with dream images that involves sensing where they are primarily felt in the body. By holding dream images in mind and carefully noticing the sensations in the various parts of the body with which the images are associated, it is possible to get a sense of how the images are grounded in the body. Image and imagination then become grounded in sensation and perception.

When the images are physically located in this way, a new sense of embodiment can emerge with a greater sense of mind body unity. We can then more easily recognise that the body informs the mind as much as the mind directs the body. Bosnak says that:

> Instead of nineteenth-century western id-to-ego colonizing models, in which a strong rational ego controls and infiltrates irrational unconscious forces, embodied imagination requires an attitude of communication. (2007, p. 25)

Candace Pert

The work of Candace Pert, who was an American neuroscientist and pharmacologist, can shed some light on the biological nature of this two way dialogue between imagination and physical symptoms. She made a breakthrough discovery when she found the "opiate receptor" or the cellular binding site for endorphins in the brain. Endorphins (endogenous or "self-made" morphine) are a type of "peptide" or chemical compound that is produced in the brain and in various other parts of the body. Peptides such as endorphins are known as "ligands" (meaning "to bind") because they bind onto cells that have appropriate receptors for them. When they bind to a cell they act as "chemical messengers" that convey information from one part of the body to another. In this way what happens in one part of the body can be shown to have a direct chemical effect on another part. "The receptor, having received a message, transmits it from the surface of the cell deep into the cell's interior, where the message can change the state of the cell dramatically" (Pert, 1997, p. 24).

Pert maintains that this kind of communication is going on in all parts of the body simultaneously. Without recourse to the nervous system the brain can alter the functioning of cells in other parts of the body just as the cells in other parts of the body can alter the functioning of the brain. She refers to the phenomenon of this whole body interaction as a "second brain". Other writers sometimes refer to this phenomenon as a "floating brain". Certain important messages are conveyed around the body in the bloodstream rather than by the nervous system. Pert's researches led her to believe "that virtually all illnesses, if not psychosomatic in foundation, (have) a definite psychosomatic component" (1997, p. 18).

She says that physiological processes are capable of triggering large changes of behaviour, physical activity, and mood. We are familiar with the fact that the psyche in turn is capable of triggering physiological changes. The example of blushing with embarrassment is an obvious case of a noticeable and immediate physiological change in response to a psychological state. When physiological changes occur with no apparent or conscious psychological correlate we need therefore to look to the unconscious to find the missing psychological aspect of a physical condition. Depth psychotherapy is a way of doing this.

One of the best ways of doing this is, in her view, to work with dreams.

> Becoming aware of your dreams is a way of eavesdropping on the conversation that is going on between psyche and soma, body and mind, of accessing levels of consciousness that are normally beyond awareness. (1997, p. 290)

She believes that strong emotions that are not consciously processed have harmful effects on our physical health. Unconscious emotions are stored in the body where they result in restricted blood flow. This deprives the frontal cortex and other organs of vital nourishment. As the body releases these withheld emotions in sleep they rise to the surface where we can experience them, as Bosnak has pointed out, in the form of feeling toned dream imagery. Experiencing these emotions consciously by dream recollection has in her view a healing effect.

When these emotional blockages are chronically stored in the body they can result in a physical weakening of organs or areas of the body concerned; making them susceptible to disease. Psychotherapy that involves revisiting and reclaiming long withheld or denied emotions is useful as a means releasing these tensions. It can allow physical disorders in the body to heal. The tissue of the body is nourished by the increased blood flow that results when the tensions of withholding are released.

Gabor Maté

The work of the Hungarian born Canadian physician Gabor Maté develops these ideas further. He uses the word "psychoneuroimmunoendocrinology" or PNI to describe his field of research. Like Pert his work explores the interrelationship between psychology and the functioning of the hormonal and neurological systems in relation to the development and healing of disease.

He points out that:

> The body's hormonal system is inextricably linked with the brain centres where emotions are experienced and interpreted. In turn, the hormonal apparatus and emotional centres are interconnected with the immune system and the nervous system ... It is impossible for any stressful stimulus, chronic or acute, to act on only one part of the super-system. What happens to one will affect all. (2003, p. 61)

He says that stress is a physiological response to a perceived threat. A perception may or may not be an accurate reading of a situation. Stress may be based on misinformation or prejudice. It therefore may or may not be a healthy adaptive response. A perceived threat triggers a chain of hormonal responses that effect the functioning of brain, nerves, pituitary, adrenal, kidney, blood vessels, connective tissues, thyroid, liver, and white blood cells as well as the interrelations between them.

Laboratory research with animals has shown that chronic stress as a result of living with a perceived threat, whether accurate or inaccurate, has a damaging effect on all of these systems and organs. These effects include enlarged adrenals, shrunken lymph organs, and ulcerated intestines (2003, p. 32).

When we are under stress hormones are released that arouse the system in preparation for fight or flight. Hormones such as adrenalin and cortisol, amongst others, arouse and regulate bodily processes such as the immune system. Blood is diverted from internal organs to the muscles while blood sugars are released for quick energy. When the mind is focused on the perceived threat, drives such as hunger and sex are forgotten. Prolonged chronic stress can lead to problems in all of these areas. Maté points out for instance that too much blood sugar will cause coma and that "an overactive immune system will soon produce chemicals that are toxic" (2003, p. 33). The body is in a state of disharmony. It is aroused but at the same time it is trying to maintain homeostasis while living with threat.

Living with this kind of emotional deadlock is harmful to the physical health of the body because:

Emotions [...] directly modulate the immune system. Studies at the US National Cancer Institute found that Natural Killer (NK) cells [...] are more active in breast cancer patients who are able to express anger, to adopt a fighting stance and who have social support. (2003, p. 61)

Maté refers to research in which the damaging results of unexpressed emotion were tangibly demonstrated.

> In one study, psychologists interviewed patients admitted to hospital for breast biopsy, without knowing the pathology results. Researchers were able to predict the presence of cancer in up to 94 percent of cases judging by psychological factors alone. (2003, p. 63)

Unconscious stress

Stress is an adaptive response to threat but what happens if stress becomes normalised or occurs below the threshold of awareness? Indeed what are the likely long term effects of a conscious and deliberate choice to embrace stress? Let us consider life in the military services. The US Department of Veteran's Affairs for example reports that up to twenty per cent of veterans from the Iraq and Afghanistan wars developed post-traumatic stress disorder (PTSD). Additionally, of the people who approached the VA for health care, some twenty-three per cent of female personnel had experienced sexual assault; while fifty-five per cent of women and twenty-eight per cent of men experienced sexual harassment (US Department of Veterans Affairs, 2014). Despite these figures we may suppose that a macho culture that to some degree normalises such stresses will ensure that issues are more likely to be unvoiced and avoided than they are to be addressed. Hence there is a high use of alcohol and tobacco in the military which serves as a coping strategy. Both the chronic stresses and the mode of coping with them are likely, over time, to have detrimental repercussions on the health of the body. In civil society there is clearly less machismo than in the military but it is not uncommon to see job placements advertised with the proviso that the candidate "must be able to work under pressure" implying that a capacity and willingness to live with chronic stress is a marketable virtue in which we might take pride.

In this way living in stress can become normalised and even idealised. It can be regarded as a part of ordinary daily living in the world. We develop the habit of ignoring the body's signals and become increasingly unconscious. We become numb and unable either to flee or fight the everyday pathological "normalities" which have aroused the stress responses.

As we have been noting throughout, there is a danger that medical and psychological therapies that aim at symptom removal will be counterproductive in terms of health. They risk more deeply embedding the physical responses to stress as they deepen unconsciousness of pathological situations which are commonly regarded as normal. In order to achieve a greater degree of health it is necessary to support a sufferer to confront or to escape a pathogenic environment.

We could consider that many of the illnesses and so called disorders that people suffer in dysfunctional and pathological systems such as workplaces, familial, social, and built environments may in fact be adaptive responses. They are adaptive in as far as they provide an exit from a damaging environment. If such stresses were to be successfully tolerated there might be deeply damaging physical and psychological repercussions. Depression, anxiety, and the gamut of recently identified and medicated "disorders" may in fact be relatively healthy means of escape from a toxic environment. Medications and therapies that alleviate or suppress such symptoms without raising awareness of the broader context in which they occur may themselves become causes of disease and disorder rather than a health giving response to them. In other words the disease may in some cases be healthier than the treatment.

Illness is not just personal

Both psychological and physical illnesses may occur when we mistake or overlook the pathology of a social system of which we are a part. If we are blind to workplace stress we may mistake the stress we feel for personal weakness as we saw in the case of Paul in Chapter Three. If we remain unaware of our stress or feel unable or unwilling to either fight or flee that which oppresses us, then both body and mind are in a state of dis-ease and are prone to illness. Just how the pathology of the social systems gets under our skin so that we manifest its illness as though it were a strictly personal matter is most readily understood if we look to the family of birth.

Family and systemic therapy explores how patterns and styles of dealing with or avoiding emotional situations are passed down the generations. There is for example a typical impact of birth order that is likely to mould a person's character. This, combined with parental expectations and wishes, means that the roles we are assigned in a family may or may not do justice to our true character. On the most basic level we can say that all birth positions come with their own potentially growthful psychological challenges and their potential pathologies. To choose but one example, it is typical that the first born in a family with younger siblings might be expected to grow up quickly while the more urgent needs of the younger siblings are being met. The oldest may learn to ignore or to deny their own dependency needs. This may lead to difficulties in emotional self-awareness and self-expression that may last a lifetime. Needs that are inadequately expressed and met might in turn lead to stress and to psychological and physical health problems.

A parent who lacks connection and ability to express their own inner emotional life is less likely to be an effective role model to their children in this regard, and so emotional issues may be passed down the generations and even amplified until consciousness is raised sufficiently to break the pattern. Family therapist Dr. Michael Kerr speaks of a "multi-generational emotional process". He says that:

> [...] physical illness, like emotional illness, is a symptom of a relationship process that extends beyond the boundaries of the individual "patient". Physical illness, in other words, is a disorder of the family emotional system [which includes] present and past generations. (Maté, 2003, p. 222)

Psychiatrist R. D. Laing wrote of the power of "attributions" to influence another person's behaviour. If a quality is attributed to us, rather than asked of us, it has a way of bypassing the ego and getting under our skin.

> The one person does not use the other merely as a hook to hang projections on. He strives to find in the other, or to induce in the other, the very embodiment of projection. The other person's collusion is required to "complement" the identity self feels compelled to sustain. One can experience a peculiar form of guilt, specific, I think, to this disjunction. If one refuses collusion, one feels guilt

for not becoming the embodiment of the complement demanded by the other for his identity. However if one does succumb, if one is seduced, one becomes estranged from one's self and is guilty thereby of self-betrayal. (1961, p. 111)

Qualities can be attributed to us when the attention of significant others is selective and our character is interpreted in ways that sustain the way they view us. It can then be very difficult even in adulthood to avoid embodying the qualities others imagine us to have. This is the case whether we are being scapegoated for a negative quality that the group of which we are a part cannot face, or if we are idealised and put on a pedestal for a quality that the projector has not yet realised in him or herself. We have seen too in the discussion of placebo and nocebo that the way our symptoms are perceived and dealt with can have a determining effect on both our physical and psychological health. Our critical skills are, of course, least developed when we are very young. Family therapists Bradley Wilson and George Edington explore the ways that children in families may be scripted by their parents to fulfil roles. These roles may have more to do with parental needs than those of the child. They say for instance that:

> [...] a special problem can arise when children of a family are— both or all- of the same sex, and one or both parental hearts had been set on having either a boy or a girl. Instead not one but two (or more) of the less wanted sex appear, and, without being aware of it, one or both of the parents, may select one of the children to stand in for that much-wanted son or daughter. In most cases it is the younger child who gets picked for this role. This is not to say that such a child will necessarily grow up as an imitation of the opposite sex, but the child often enters adulthood with exaggerated self-doubts as to whether or not he or she is adequately living up to the gender and sex-role stereotypes which our society still assigns to males and females. (1981, p. 276)

The family system can have an influence that may lead to the creation of a false sense of self. It thus sets up the conditions for unconscious stress and possibly damaging consequences for both psychological and physical health. In addition to the above, the family may ascribe to us any number of roles which may have little to do with our actual authentic identity. Perhaps we are induced to express anger on behalf of others who cannot or dare not do so. We may be given the role of the impulsive one or the sensitive one, the peacemaker, the troublemaker, or any other of innumerable scripts which we may enact at the cost of discovering and expressing our authentic self.

These false roles create dis-ease, they lead us into conflict with our inner nature. Diseases produce symptoms and problems in managing a life that is not in accord with our authentic selves. They block our path, they force new behaviours upon us. Our vulnerabilities open us up to new possibilities for self-realisation. We can no longer cope in the manner of our old "familiar" self.

The individual as a carrier of social dis-ease

We have seen in the case of Paul in Chapter Three how workplace pressures can create or contribute to stress which in turn can engender disease. We have noted how the medical establishment in the form of the *Diagnostic and Statistical Manual* (DSM) with its language of personal "disorders" can turn our attention away from the social dimensions of illness. It can focus treatment on supposedly disordered individuals while allowing pathogenic environments and social systems to remain unnoticed, unchallenged, and unaltered. A stressed and weakened workforce or a populace propped up by costly and often unnecessary pharmaceutical treatments that can be shown to work little if any better than placebo remedies can make it possible to overlook the social dimension of disease.

The Austrian philosopher Ivan Illich held that in this way the medical establishment can be said to:

> [...] mystify and [...] expropriate the power of the individual to heal himself and to shape his or her environment [...]. Such medicine is but a device to convince those who are sick and tired of society that it is they who are ill, impotent, and in need of technical repair. (1976, p. 16)

A psychotherapy that focuses exclusively on the individual can be part of the problem of ill health rather than a part of the solution. If psychotherapy is to be more potent as a healing agent it must look beyond the strictly personal dimensions of healing. Psychotherapists sometimes fight shy of the social and environmental dimensions of illness. Some psychotherapists see references to such "external" factors as an avoidance of personal issues. They do not see these considerations as a way of deepening the apparently personal into the broader and deeper collective psychology of which the personal is but a part.

The psychoanalyst Ralph Greenson caught himself doing exactly this in relation to one of his patients who was suffering from stomach ulcers and depression. When the patient referred to political views with which Greenson disagreed, he responded in a way that suggested that the patient needed to explore his inner world more deeply.

> He [...] told me that whenever he said anything favorable about a Republican politician, I always asked for associations. On the other hand, whenever he said anything hostile about a Republican, I remained silent. Whenever he had a kind word for Roosevelt, I said nothing. Whenever he attacked Roosevelt, I would ask who did Roosevelt remind him of, as though I was out to prove that hating Roosevelt was infantile.
>
> I was taken aback because I had been completely unaware of this pattern. Yet, at the moment the patient pointed it out, I had to agree that I had done precisely that, albeit unknowingly. We then went to work on why he felt the need to try to swallow my political views. This turned out to be his way of ingratiating himself with me. This proved indigestible and lowered his self-esteem, leading to the ulcer symptoms and the depressiveness. (1967, p. 273)

Greenson became aware that his interventions or lack of them invalidated his patient's outward political views by suggesting that they were unconscious unresolved personal issues. As is the case with the tendency to speak in terms of psychiatric "disorders", he took the emphasis off the patient's legitimate response to the world about him. Unaware of his own prejudices he inadvertently reinforced his patient's symptoms. The result was that the patient more deeply embodied his symptoms when the therapeutic aim was to move toward health.

Archetypal psychologist James Hillman in his book (co-written with Michael Ventura) and tellingly titled *We've Had 100 Years of Psychotherapy and the World is Getting Worse,* offers examples of how the profession can become entrapped in an exclusively personalistic view of illness.

He says of psychiatry that it is caught in the belief that depression and physical symptoms without identifiable causes are "endogenic" or self-caused.

> We used to believe, and studies "showed", that stress came from inside the patient's psychic field of personal relations: death of a loved one, moving to another house, divorce or breakup, bankruptcy, failure, or being fired. These were said to be the shocks that the soul and body couldn't easily take and caused "stress" reactions.
>
> But now new studies "show" stress arises largely from the "irritations of daily life", which I take to mean again the aesthetic disorders of the environment, such as racism, noise, crowding, traffic, air quality, crime fears, police cars, violence fears, legal threats, hypercommunication (too much info, keeping up) breakdowns and frustrations in the school systems, taxpaying, bureaucracy, hospitals, and making ends meet. (1992, p. 81)

Hillman describes how the social and physical environment itself intrudes into our personal psychic space. Stress is not generated from within in this case but has a social and environmental origin. Can a person be said to be disordered when they become ill as a result of the chronic stresses related to the environment in which they live?

The sickened psyche

The situation can seem clearer and less subtle when we experience the results of environmental disorder in a manifestly physical condition such as for example the effects of environmental poisoning from tetraethyl lead or lead emissions from car exhausts.

In the 1920s lead began to be added to petroleum in order to improve the engine performance and fuel economy of cars. Between the mid-1970s and the early 2000s it was gradually phased out in most countries. This was due, in the main, to public health concerns. The toxic nature of lead affects all organs and functions of the body to varying degrees. Patients suffering from such poisoning may present with a wide range of symptoms including, amongst others, effects on the nervous, gastrointestinal, reproductive systems, and kidney complaints. It is known to be particularly damaging to children and to unborn babies. Other research indicates that it is strongly suspected to have psychological and behavioural effects, and to be linked with criminality (Monbiot, 2013). However, to "successfully" treat the patient's illness without also addressing the pathologies that underpin it, is at best a limited kind of healing.

On a superficial level we can say that the underlying "cause" of the poisoning is lead emissions. Yet it is important to remember that the decision to remove lead from petrol was not based on the discovery of its harmful effects. These were perfectly well known prior to its introduction in the 1920s. Indeed "soon after production began in 1922 in Bayway, New Jersey, USA an outbreak of acute neuropsychiatric disease appeared among workers, 80% of whom developed convulsions and five died" (Scott, 2011).

Nor was lead ever necessary in order to achieve the beneficial effects on car engine performance. Ethanol or alcohol was already known to do the same job just as effectively and was low in toxicity, widely available, and inexpensive (Kitman, 2000). Tetraethyl lead was preferred because it could not only be produced in sufficient quantities to meet the demand but also because it was a manufactured process that could be profitably patented (Kitman, 2000). We can imagine that the individual shareholders in this enterprise were more likely to feel the financial benefits of this arrangement and less likely to live beside busy urban streets where they would experience the toxic effects of the poisoning. However, we must remember too that all of those in society who hold savings bonds or pensions may themselves be responsible as inadvertent investors in such environmental sickness.

Lead poisoning is not best understood as a strictly personal or physical condition. It has social and psychological underpinnings. It says as much about the pathology of the social and psychological environment in which it occurs as it says about the physical state of the individual who manifests the symptom. "Psyche" means "breath". A sickened atmosphere is a sickened psyche.

Nor is this simply a matter of recent history on which we can afford to passively reflect. Amongst the many atmospheric pollutants from which we suffer today are the effects of diesel exhaust emissions. The World Health Organisation classifies these as carcinogens belonging in the same category as mustard gas and asbestos. These are known to cause lung and bladder cancer. In 2014 London's main shopping street, Oxford Street, distinguished itself when it was shown to have the world's highest levels of toxic nitrogen dioxide, which comes from diesel engines (Bertini, 2014).

We can argue that to truly heal such a condition, like a disease caused by environmental poisoning, we also need as individuals to address the poisonous underlying psychological, social, and political issues that support it. In this way we see that the disease from which we suffer is a part of our calling; a voice of the personal daimon demanding a response from us. It reminds us that we are members of a community and an integral part of the greater world that we inhabit. The disease awakens us to a task required of us in, by, and for the world.

Individual and social health are in this way inextricably tied on both the physical and psychological level. Unhealthy social and environmental stresses that come to our attention in the form of physical or psychological illness need to be raised to consciousness. They may perhaps then be healthily fought, fled from, or responded to creatively. Psychotherapy can help us to come into conscious relationship with external stressors rather than be unconsciously absorbed in pathogenic collective norms. We can then take Illich's point. Mainstream medicine on its own may "expropriate the power of the individual to heal himself and to shape his or her environment".

In this way social mores change and evolve. Yesterday's stressful punishable criminal offence such as homosexual acts, for instance, can become today's socially approved and accepted behaviour blessed by the sacrament of marriage. While the relaxed use of yesterday's children's cough remedy marketed by the Bayer Drug Company until 1912 under the brand name "Heroin" has become today's criminal offence.

CHAPTER NINE

Anima mundi—the world psyche

The French philosopher Maurice Merleau-Ponty recognised that our experiences are not exclusively our own. He said that, "It is not just I that sees and hears but also my flesh that belongs to the flesh of the world that sees and hears" (1968, p. 142). We have seen that matters we need to address in our lives for the sake of becoming more whole and healthy may come to our attention in the form of physical or psychological symptoms and/or illness. These may be manifestly personal in character but at the same time rooted in psychological and physical processes that encompass more than just us. They can draw our attention to the fact that our personal issues are a part of a bigger pattern. We may be struck by the fact that we are a part of a family dynamic that needs to be raised to consciousness in order to be healed. Conditions that we sometimes assume are strictly personal may in fact originate and be fuelled by others. We may be entrenched in patterns that began with our ancestors. To the extent that we have not appreciated this we might even feel that those ancestors continue to "haunt" us with their poorly adapted assumptions, values, and life style choices. We may continue to unconsciously perpetuate these patterns and behaviours until we ourselves are confronted with a crisis in the form of physical or psychological illness.

We can see that the same dynamic is present in social situations such as the workplace. There, our problems are not necessarily best understood as being solely of our own making. The stresses which build up when we strive to adapt to the demands of an unhealthy work, social, or family environment may become the trigger for personal symptoms and disease. Sometimes it is only then that we recognise the need for fight or flight, whatever the personal cost may be. So too we have seen that we can subscribe to social norms such as driving cars and contributing to personal pension schemes unconscious of the fact that we are contributing to toxicity in the environment until it is brought to our personal attention in the form of physical illness. Even then we may use mainstream medicine as a way of suppressing this potentially emerging awareness. Such lack of awareness implies a lack of response to problems that grow increasingly acute until they reach epidemic proportions. Then on a personal or collective level we reach a crisis, a crossroad, a turning point where we are obliged to take another direction.

We are all a part of the community of human beings. With varying degrees of awareness we participate in the collective pathologies of our time. We have little choice about this. However the story does not end there. We are also a part of the much greater fabric of life itself. We have noted that this awareness has been voiced by insightful thinkers such as Albert Einstein and Thich Nhat Hahn. Jung expressed it in this way.

> [...] life is a kind of unit, [...] it is really a continuum and meant to be as it is, namely, all one tissue in which things live through or by means of each other. Therefore trees cannot be without animals, nor animals without plants, and perhaps animals cannot be without man, and man cannot be without animals and plants—and so on. The whole thing is one tissue and so no wonder that all the parts function together, as the cells in our bodies function together, because they are of the same living continuum. (2002, p. 207)

Jung held the view expressed by Plato that the world itself has a soul or psyche. He considered that the psyche is not something that appeared spontaneously from nowhere when life has evolved to a certain degree of complexity. It is not the by-product of a complicated brain structure but is instead a part of the very bedrock, the fabric of the world. Indeed it is integral to the very cosmos of which our world is but a part.

He subscribed to an ancient conception known in Latin as the *Anima Mundi* and in Greek as the *Psyche tou Kosmou*, meaning "the soul of the world".

Sapient earth

To be "human" is to be "of the earth" or in effect of the "humus". We are the "earthy ones" or the "earth born"; just as the Biblical Adam was created "from the dust of the ground" (1970, p. 2). To be homo-sapiens is, as we discussed earlier, to be a part of the earth that is "sapient" or wise. This idea of an animate or ensouled world is one that can be found in many cultures. For example the aboriginal people of Australia regard themselves as being "born into" a totemic identity with an aspect of the natural world. This might be a plant or an animal or another phenomenon of the natural world such as water, or the wind (Cowan, 1992, p. 39). In other words an aboriginal Australian would regard him or herself as more than just a human being. He or she would feel themselves also to be that element of what we would call "external" reality which is their totem.

The totemic identity is determined before birth by the spirit of the specific place of conception. The individual is considered to have a specific affinity with a geographical place of which he or she is believed to be an embodiment. It is not so much the case that the person has an intimate tie with the world in this way. It is more the case that the individual is believed to be a part of the very fabric of the world, a part of the continuum of that of which the world is made. Jung felt this was true in his own day and age. Jung expressed the view that to be born in a geographical place was at a profound level to be an embodiment of the "spirit" of that place. This is the case despite ones ethnic or cultural heritage. He said that:

> There is an x and a y in the air and the soil of a country, which slowly permeate and assimilate him to the type of the aboriginal inhabitant, even to the point of slightly remodelling his physical features [...] these subtle indications [...] sometimes [...] lurk in the lines of his face, sometimes in his gestures, his facial expression, the look in his eyes, and sometimes in his psyche, that shines forth through the transparent veil of his body. (1964, p. 510)

Jung here proposes that we are a child of the land of our birth as well as that of our parents and culture. He suggests that we are born from animate forces within the fabric of the environment around us or perhaps more accurately the environment of which we are a part. His views beg the question as to whether or not there is a sense in which there can be such a thing as a psychology of place and if so what its influence and significance to those who visit or inhabit a particular place might be.

The Australian Aboriginal tradition is a non-literate one. Before the arrival of Europeans, much of the tribal knowledge was passed on in the form of songs. In order to navigate ones way around a vast continent which over great areas has only limited survival resources it was necessary to know where to find food and water as well as landmarks and boundaries. The mythology of the land and of the heavens was recounted in the form of traditional ceremonial songs. These enabled people to travel safely over vast distances (Norris, 2014). The routes indicated by such songs became known by Europeans as "songlines" or "dreaming tracks".

David Abram suggests that knowledge of the landscape recounted in a preliterate society such as this suggests a more intimate involvement with the land than is easy for us to imagine. He suggests that there is synaesthesia at work whereby for them to visually and sensually perceive the land is at the same time to "hear" its voice. The song is experienced as the voice of the land. The land speaks.

This idea is less obscure if we look to our own experience with the written word. Written words, after all, are simply marks on a piece of paper. To a non-literate person they are meaningless and dead. Yet to us they speak. In a sense we "hear" with our eyes. These mute marks on paper can awaken and inform us with their sometimes vivid stories, their rhythms, humour, imagery, nuance, and information. Such may be the experience of the Aboriginal or the preliterate to the landscape itself. Perhaps too we have purchased our literacy at the expense of this more immediate sensitivity and connection with our environment.

The writer and journalist Bruce Chatwin recounts an incident in which he was driving through the Outback of Australia in the company of an Aboriginal man who suddenly became extremely agitated when they crossed a part of his songline.

> His eyes rolled wildly over the rocks, the cliffs, the palms, the water.
> His lips moved at the speed of a ventriloquist's and, through them,
> came a rustle: the sound of wind through branches. (1987, p. 293)

The driver recognised what was happening and slowed the vehicle down to a walking pace. He realised that the man was recounting the song of the land at the speed of a jeep being driven across the Outback. When he slowed the vehicle down to a walking pace the man smiled happily and the sound he made became "a lovely melodious swishing" as the story unfolded at a human pace.

In a world of motorways and jet travel it is easy for us to feel estranged and disconnected from a land that has for us in the main become demythologised and "unsung". We are no longer present enough or receptive enough to hear the voice of the land. We have to a great extent forgotten its myths. Mistaking the "imaginal" for the "imaginary" we easily overlook the power of geographical place and the imagery it provokes. Psychotherapy can, as we have seen, contribute to this process of personalising psychological forces that belong to the environment. "We've had a hundred years of psychotherapy and the world is getting worse", said Hillman and Ventura.

Jung held that the psyche is fundamentally "chthonic" or "of the earth". To be unconscious of this aspect of the psyche was in his view a grave danger.

> The facts of nature cannot in the long run be violated. Penetrating and seeping through everything like water, they will undermine any system that does not take account of them, and sooner or later they will bring about its downfall. (1941, p. 109)

Let us consider then how we might deepen our awareness of psychological processes to include this chthonic element with the aim of attending to a more comprehensive wholing or healing.

A psychology of place

As psychotherapists we can easily imagine the process of unconsciously projecting personal issues into the surrounding environment. We may see it as our psychotherapeutic task to help others to reclaim personal responsibility for those conditions that they incorrectly imagine to be happening to them. But what if there is two-way traffic here? What if we were to entertain, as Jung suggests, the possibility that our basic nature (the chthonic psyche) projects its contents into us? Then our task must be to "take account" of this. We must look to and recognise what it is in the world, in the surrounding environment, that demands or draws our attention. We must aim to find a conscious and creative way to admit and to express those energies; lest they, as do other unconscious psychic contents, sabotage us and undermine our health.

American psychologist Craig Chaquist puts the challenge this way.

> When people inhabit a particular place, its features inhabit their psychological field, in effect becoming extended facets of their selfhood. The more they repress this local, multifaceted sense of environmental presence, the likelier its features will reappear unconsciously as symbolic, animated forces seething from within and from without. (2007, p. 7)

Is it possible that the living environment that we inhabit is capable of projecting its content into us? As we have seen to be the case with the family and the workplace, if we do not recognise the psychological impact of qualities that are projected onto us we are likely to feel pathogenic stress and/or to embody those qualities and act them out.

Chalquist writes of how he felt that he had been unconsciously infected by the spirit of his home town of San Diego in California. At a time when he was doing a sociological study of the town he found himself becoming depressed. Although he did not understand why he should be feeling depressed he attributed this to his relationship. He experienced what he describes as a puzzling and growing sense of "caginess and guardedness" with his partner. It was not until he had an impressive dream that he was able to reframe his feelings in a way that made more sense to him. The woman with whom he found himself in the dream was not his lover as he expected her to be, but instead she startlingly identified herself to him as "San Diego". In the light of San Diego's geographical situation of being a border town with many illegal migrants and a major naval base his "cagey" and "guarded" feelings made a great deal more sense to him. His further study of the "environmental presence" of the city, its "story", its history, and sociology, enabled him to relate more consciously to his location. This enabled him to better distinguish feelings picked up in the atmosphere of this specific place from those that belonged to his human relationships.

Is it more than poetic licence to say that a town or geographical place can have a character, a personality, a psychology, a spirit, a soul? And if somehow this can be said to be the case what effect does a particular place have upon those who live in it or visit it? Perhaps like any relationship to another human being or an animal, some will get on better with a particular place than will others. We will all have different impressions of the spirit of place depending on what we bring to it and what we expect and want from it. Like any relationship it will also depend on what the place brings to and requires from us. Stories and myths of place are built up by the experience of its friends, foes, lovers and its workmates. As with people, places too have developmental traumas, failures and successes, strengths and weaknesses. To attend to, and to deepen relationship to place we can ask what it is that individuals and places can offer one another.

Penwith dreaming

With this in mind let us take a look at Penwith. Penwith is that part Great Britain which is at the most extreme south-western end of the English county of Cornwall (or Kernow). It is at the end of a long peninsula jutting "hornlike" into the Atlantic Ocean (Kernow means "horn" in the old Celtic Cornish language). Geographically it is an ancient land composed largely of granite rock that once formed the roots of a great range of mountains. In parts of the county you can find serpentine rock that has condensed from the mantle of the earth. It is rich in minerals, particularly tin, which made it a favoured trading destination in the ancient world. If, as legend has it, Christ once visited the British Isles it is most likely he would have come to Penwith.

In Penwith you can find the remains of ancient civilisations. Some of the existing structures predate the building of the Egyptian pyramids. The landscape is dotted with ancient monuments such as stone circles, holy wells, fortifications, Celtic crosses, burial chambers, and mysterious womblike underground chambers known as "fogous". Penwith and its offshore islands are as near to the setting sun as it is possible to be in England. The tomb builders apparently felt that it was the natural place to commune with the dead and the spirits of the ancestors.

Penwith was also the last outpost of the land of Kernow to lose its native Celtic language and with it, its direct line of continuity with its past. The last born speaker is known to have died in 1777. With a very few exceptions Kernowek or Cornish was an unwritten language. This suggests perhaps that the voice of the land may have spoken louder and more recently here than it did in the rest of England. The widespread illiteracy of the Cornish speakers ensured that there was a vigorous oral tradition of myth and legends of the land. Many of these stories were rescued from oblivion in the nineteenth century by such mythographers as Robert Hunt and William Bottrell. Thanks to them we still have a lively record of the voice of the land and the panoply of legendary and supernatural figures that were believed to inhabit it. Indeed in parts of Penwith the stories of place are numerous enough to constitute a sort of Cornish "story line" that could be told or heard in situ at a walking pace.

Ancient energies

This ancient charged atmosphere of Penwith can on occasions be sensed in extraordinary ways. Take for example the case of Penwith resident, writer, and Professor Alan Bleakley who at one time lived near one of Penwith's 6000 year old burial chambers or "quoits". He writes of an occasion when he recalled a dream. He says he was told in the dream that he should visit the quoit at four a.m. on the day of the winter solstice. He followed the instruction of his dream and headed out in the dead of night through "pelting rain" to arrive at the quoit at the appointed hour. He says that at that moment there was a "peel of thunder" and "sheet lightening lit the sky". He heard a disembodied man's voice behind him say an unfamiliar word "Karas!" It was not until the next Easter that he again encountered the word "karas". He was at a conference where he learned that the term referred to an Egyptian method of embalming a dead body in the expectation that there would be a rebirth in the spirit world (1984, pp. 1–2).

Take too the example of Kenneth, a Penwith man in his fifties who also had a significant dream. In his case the dream was one of having inadvertently discovered an underground chamber. Inside he was amazed to find what he took to be group of gigantic ancient stone figures sitting in the vast dark space as though in deep silent meditation. As his eyes gradually became accustomed to the darkness he became aware that the figures were in fact not made of stone at all. They were actually living breathing ancestral beings who meditated beneath the land. Despite being disturbed the awesome figures were not hostile to the intruder but instead offered him instruction.

In response to the dream Kenneth decided to visit in actuality one of these ancient tombs, to sleep, and to dream there. After having dreamt and on his return from the tomb he tripped over a rock, fell, and broke a bone. He also suffered a concussion and a torn retina in one eye. He was discovered on the path by a passer-by. He was still in a kind of trance state and was unable to account for himself. His injuries were shocking and traumatic yet nevertheless they echoed rituals that are believed by some to have been performed in these ancient places. The chambers were regarded as places where the living could meet and commune with ancestral spirits provided they had first been contacted by the spirit world in a dream. There, in the dark of the interior behind a wall of stone were the mortal remains of ancestors. In preparation for the encounter initiates were sometimes induced into a trance state in order to improve their receptivity to the voices of the spirits. In South American cultures, for example, the preparation to encounter the spirits of the dead would include a period of fasting followed by drinking copious quantities of tobacco juice or other narcotics regarded to be "magical substances". In some initiations in which the dead were to be encountered the candidate was prepared for the encounter by first being beaten unconscious by the master (Eliade, 1964, pp. 83–84). Sometimes it was said that a bone was deliberately broken. This symbolised a ritual death or the breaking of an old way of being. Traditionally it was believed that the initiate would then be reassembled or reborn as an intermediary between the spiritual and earthly worlds. With regard to the Kenneth's eye injury we can note that in mythology a figure such as the Teutonic god Odin or Woden, was obliged first to sacrifice an eye in order that he might gain the "third eye" of wisdom (Graves, 1959, p. 261).

We can see that both in Alan Bleakley's and in Kenneth's experiences there are echoes of archaic beliefs and rituals that may well have been familiar to the tomb builders. Such spontaneous experiences encountered today in an animated landscape evoke and revive a sense of our long forgotten mysterious connection with the spirits of the earth, those serpentine Asklepian energies that bring healing up from the underworld into the light of consciousness.

The black and the white

Cornwall is today England's poorest county. After more than 2000 years its mining industry has collapsed and died. The last working mine closed in 1998. The county is today strewn with the picturesque overgrown ruins of abandoned industrial buildings. The bleakly beautiful despoiled landscape remains largely denuded of its trees. Only patches of hidden woodland with lichen covered trees that benefit from the unpolluted Atlantic air suggest how the preindustrial landscape may have looked. Its other two main industries of agriculture and fishing are today not profitable enough to sustain a large population. Cornwall relies heavily today on the tourism industry. Its lovely golden sand surfing beaches, hidden coves, and its wild landscapes draw people from Britain and abroad. It is a favoured location for those seeking a healthier alternative lifestyle as well as for artists and writers to work. It is also a popular place for stressed city folk to retire or to own a second home. It is hard for local people to find work other than that which is poorly paid and seasonal. Owning property is difficult for the low paid. Consequently many young people leave the county to pursue their careers elsewhere perpetuating the now long standing tradition of the Cornish diaspora.

The Cornish national flag is the cross of Saint Piran. Piran was a sixth century Cornish abbot who is now widely accepted as the patron saint of Cornwall. He is believed to have brought Christianity to Cornwall from across the sea in Ireland. It is a stark white cross on a background of black. It is said by some to represent the bright gleaming deposits of tin hidden in the black earth. The black and the white could also be seen to suggest a kind of splitting that is perhaps characteristic of Cornish psychology. Certainly for the tourist or visitor Cornwall hides many dark secrets. Take the Penwith town of St. Ives for instance; famous for its wonderful light, beautiful golden sand beaches, and subtropical vegetation. The town is built on a hill which is on a peninsula which is itself upon the Penwith peninsula. It is surrounded by an often Mediterranean blue sea. The golden sand beneath the clear water reflects the light in shades of turquoise. Visually, it is as near as the British Isles can get to a Greek fishing village with its quaint higgledy-piggledy buildings and narrow cobbled streets. It remains today an important magnet for artists and has been home to such internationally acclaimed figures as the sculptor Barbara Hepworth and the potter Bernard Leach. For most of the year it throngs with visitors; some of whom leave loving tributes expressing their gratitude and appreciation of the town's remarkable and inspiring beauty on memorial benches by the sea when they die. That is the white.

But what of the black? What is it that remains unseen and overlooked by the tourist board? Let us begin with the land itself. St. Ives is radioactive. This is naturally produced radiation from the granite rock below the town. Marie Curie performed her early experiments with radium taken from the Trenwith Mine in St. Ives. The ore, known as uraninite or pitchblende, was regarded as waste when it was mined and was therefore dumped onto the hillside beside the mine. Later some 694 tons of uranium ore was taken from these dumps in St. Ives. The mine site now serves as the town's main bus terminal and a car park (Dangerous Laboratories, 2014). A little way along St. Ives Bay you will find the ruins of an arsenic works. Arsenic was regarded as a valuable soil improver in the early nineteenth century. Further along still you will find the ruined buildings of the National Explosives Works which was established in 1888 to supply both the mines and the Royal Navy with dynamite. The twentieth century then offered this coast a chemical weapons factory at Nancekuke which you will find a few miles further to the east. Here in the 1950s some fifteen tons of Sarin were produced and stored for many years to test its shelf life. In 2014 the pressure group *Surfers against Sewage* protested at South West Water's frequent discharges of untreated human sewage into the bay which is popular with bathers and surfers (Ferris, 2014).

As for the town itself, it is literally "undermined" with the abandoned and sometimes uncharted mineshafts of the tinners. In St. Ives today houses sometimes crack and sink, and car parks open into sinkholes that unexpectedly appear. The beautiful beaches are also an after effect of the mining industry. Over the centuries the rocky shores have been covered with the spoils of the mining industry deposited from the nearby Red River. In the past it and the sand it deposited were indeed red with the iron oxide contained within the spoils. And the quaint pretty houses? Many of them when built were equipped with pilchard cellars. Fishing was the business of St. Ives and the town would have reeked of fish.

Historically too St. Ives has a good deal of darkness. Take the story of John Payne for instance. John Payne was the "portreeve" of St. Ives (a kind of harbour master) at the time of the Cornish Prayer Book Rebellion in 1549. At that time the Cornish took exception to the recently deceased King Henry VIII's destruction of the Catholic Church and his establishment of the Church of England. However, the rebellion was not solely concerned with purely spiritual matters. Amongst other factors the Cornish took exception to the matter of being obliged to conduct the liturgy in English rather than in Latin. Latin, though it was not understood by most churchgoers, was an accepted universal language for Christian worship. English however was a foreign language to the Cornish. An obligation to use this foreign language represented a threat to the Cornish national identity and its customs. John Payne accepted a lunch invitation at a St. Ives Inn from the visiting English Provost Marshal (an officer in charge of the military police). The provost instructed him to arrange that a gallows be erected while they dined. After the meal he decreed that John Payne be hanged for being a "busy rebel". John Payne became one of many influential Cornishmen to be ruthlessly murdered by the English at that time.

Nor is it widely known that the Cornish were the victims of the Barbary slave trade which thrived between the sixteenth and the nineteenth centuries. The Penwith town of Mousehole was one of a number of coastal towns to be raided by African slave traders. Captives were forced to work on pirate ships or destined to be sold as European slaves in North Africa.

Cornwall is in some respects a beleaguered nation. Historically it has been invaded by outsiders and murderously robbed of its language. As with other oppressed nationalities and ethnic groups, there can be a kind of passive resignation and resentment. This can be superficially mistaken for an acceptance of the status quo. The sometimes unconscious anger that underlies this resignation has the potential to erupt into an angry demand for self-determination. This has been the case in other Celtic nations such as Ireland, Scotland, and Wales. Today in Cornwall there can be a mostly hidden but understandable degree of hostility toward incomers who's greater prosperity allows them privileges such as owning property that the locals themselves and their children cannot afford. In the 1970s and 1980s this feeling came to a head in neighbouring Wales when a group known as Meibion Glyndŵr (the sons of Glyndŵr) sustained a campaign of arson attacks on holiday homes. The group in effect swapped roles and oppressed those whom they felt to be their oppressors. As these issues become more widely discussed, there is some evidence today that Cornwall may be rediscovering its buried but energising warrior energy and expressing this in creative ways in order to initiate change for the better.

The mermaid of Zennor

How does this proposed local characteristic of black and white splitting affect those who encounter it? Let us be guided by a myth belonging to the village of Zennor near St. Ives. The myth is related by William Bottrell in the Cornish dialect.

> It tells of the occasional mysterious appearance of an extraordinarily beautiful woman at church services in Zennor. The Zennor folk admired her fine singing voice and were mystified that the woman retained her beauty over scores of years, yet none knew "whence she came or whither she went". She showed some interest in a young man in the congregation named Mathey Trewella. He was bold enough to follow her from church one day and the pair was never seen again.
>
> However, word soon spread that a mermaid had been spotted by sailors in a nearby cove. She rose from the waters and requested that the sailors lift their anchor as it was blocking the door to her "submarine abode". The local people concluded that it was she who had enticed Mathey to her underwater home. To commemorate these events they had her likeness "carved in holy-oak, which may still be seen." (1873, pp. 288–289)

And indeed it may still be seen in the twenty-first century inside the church at Zennor. Although this is to us clearly a fanciful story this was not necessarily always the case. It is worth noting the remarkable fact that until the nineteenth century an English law still claimed that "all mermaids found in British waters" were the property of the Crown (Holmes, 1974, p. 228).

On one level we have the story of a young man lured to his doom by the feminine principle in her inferior form as a mermaid. Although she is alluring she is also at least half unconscious as she lives for the most part out of sight beneath the waters. Outwardly it might express a fear of the power of women. While more symbolically it might indicate the dangers of an undeveloped feeling function. A man who is out of touch with his feelings is in danger of being unexpectedly overwhelmed by them. In this case it is even to the point that he never re-emerges.

But it is also a story of place. It happens specifically in Zennor, in Penwith, in Cornwall, and in Britain as well as in the world. Bearing in mind what we have said about the exquisite charms of nearby St. Ives we may see a modern parable. We are in a place that has the power to charm and seduce both the visitor and the unwary migrant. The obvious beauties conceal a mostly unacknowledged darkness. Stephen, a recent migrant to St. Ives intuited these dangers in a dream shortly before settling into his new home.

> I open a letter from the estate agent. It contains a warning about the house we are purchasing in St. Ives. It is apparently only a few hundred yards away from a pub called "The Spear" which is notorious as one of the most dangerous pubs in the world. It was written about in a famous novel. Someone had been stabbed through the heart there.

For many migrants the opportunity to live in this beautiful part of the world represents the fulfilment of a dream. But beware of the curse of having your dream come true. If you can't be happy when you have everything you wish for, then you do most certainly have a problem. In this case he had in his dream correctly intuited problems that were soon to surface both in his relationship and in his work life. Stephen quickly became disillusioned as he struggled with a stressful, disappointing, and ultimately intolerable work situation. He felt as if the skills that he brought to his work were resented by his colleagues more than they were valued or appreciated. He felt rejected and marginalised. His job options were few; living as he now did in England's poorest county at the end of a peninsula with an underdeveloped infrastructure and poor transport links. In his case, alternative work necessitated distant travel. While he struggled in these ways his wife struggled with her own stress and succumbed to her tendency to overuse alcohol. Here in this sunset land of the ancestors and of endings both the relationship and job ended. The dream came to its end. He confronted a life challenge that could have pulled him under and submerged him, never again to resurface as it did Mathey Trewella. His dis-illusion required that he make a new beginning. Stephen was resourceful enough to do this once he had achieved a fuller awareness of the shadow of Penwith life.

That of which we are unconscious we are destined to enact. "If you bring forth what is within you, what you bring forth will save you. If you do not bring forth what is within you, what you do not bring forth will destroy you." But what if that of which you are unconscious is not strictly yours or only yours? What if it belongs at least in part to others and to the culture and spirit of the land that you inhabit? In Stephen's case the pain of his disillusion was all the more acute as a result of his unrealistically high expectations; although his dream suggested that he had an unconscious intuitive appreciation of what was to come. But it may not only have been a matter of his idealised expectations. He may also have had the perfectly realistic expectation that his contribution to the workplace would be valued and appreciated rather than resented by his colleagues. Perhaps there was a reversal of roles in which those who felt oppressed by outsiders had themselves become the oppressors of an outsider. The more unconscious such an issue is the less it is subject to ego control and the more likely it is to be acted out in a destructive way. Had the mermaid, the beautiful seductress, had her part in pulling him under?

In order to live in a healthy relationship with a geographical place it may be necessary both as natives and as incomers to know its story, its mythology, its psychology, and its spirit if we are not to unconsciously merge with it. Then we risk becoming an embodiment of its issues. Stephen found himself feeling the dark side of what many Cornish people sometimes feel; marginalised, unvalued, misused, overlooked, forgotten, resigned, and resentful. Like Cornwall itself Stephen needed to recreate his life in a fuller consciousness of the psychology and spirit of place.

In order to be whole or healthy the black and white need to be in balance. When we strive toward "wellbeing" rather than "health" as we have defined them, our denial of pathology can create tension and dis-ease. This principle is better understood in some Eastern cultures as we noted in the Chinese "Good luck, bad luck, who's to say?" story. The principle is represented visually in the Chinese Taoist Yin-Yang symbol. Here a circle is divided by an S-shaped line. One segment is black and the other is white. These represent respectively *yin* and *yang*, or the female and male principles. Each contains a circular dot or "seed" of the other colour at its centre. The Taoist image shows these principles in a dynamic fluid relationship. They are seen as complementary and interdependent in nature rather than as oppositional. Each principle contains the other within it. Each can only exist by virtue of the existence of its complementary opposite. In the light we find a shadow. In the dark we find the potential for enlightenment.

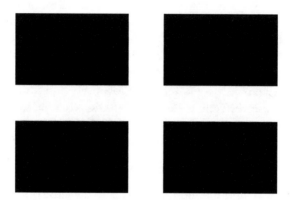

The Cornish flag of St. Piran.

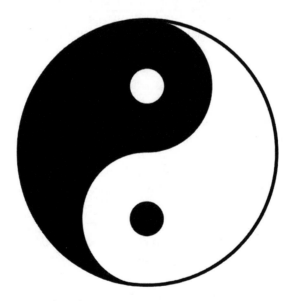

The Chinese Taoist yin-yang symbol.

CHAPTER TEN

Dancing with the devil

With illness, as with human relationships, problems and difficulties are not always best dealt with by means of denial, suppression, and combat. We have explored the ambivalent, paradoxical, daimonic nature of illness. Good luck, bad luck, who's to say? The curse of illness is sometimes felt in retrospect to be a blessing in disguise as has been attested by many of the writers to whom we have referred.

We've noted too that some medics today advocate a certain degree of tolerance and acceptance of less than perfect wellbeing. They suggest that we might still consider ourselves to be well so long as we have the ability to adapt and self-manage our physical and psychological limitations and shortcomings. The arguments presented in the preceding chapters propose that there is still further that we can go. Perhaps we can even find meaning and value in our health issues. Illness may sometimes stop us from following destructive habitual patterns; stop us from doing what is not in the best interests of our health and development. Illness may force or oblige us to change our way of being by putting us in touch with feelings and capacities that we have ignored or overlooked. If we can find meaning and value in the new experience that we have to face we may profit from our adversity. We have proposed that psychotherapy or "attending to the soul" is a way of nurturing this very process.

If illness is indeed "daimonic" as has been argued, all three positions are correct and without contradiction. Illness can at times be experienced as a curse, it can sometimes be accepted and tolerated, and in some instances it can offer opportunities for life enhancing self-discovery, change, insight, and enlightenment. Much, but not all, depends on how we respond to our condition. Arguably a healthy response will be a mixture of all three of these positions. There will be moments of opposition and fight, times of tolerance and acceptance, and occasions when we feel gratitude and appreciation for the life lessons we learn when we are ill.

We must in a sense learn to "dance" with the apparent demon of illness. In order to deal with illness in a heathy way we must find the willingness to engage, respond, and interact with it in the hopes of redeeming our suffering. We need to develop our capacity to see beyond the metaphors of war and repression if we are to discover the angel that stands behind or is hidden within the apparent devil that confronts us. This is the message of the *yin-yang* symbol, of Jesus in the gospel of Thomas, of St. Theresa of Avila, and it is why Abu Hamed al Ghazali says that illnesses are the servants of God that he sends to his friends.

If we can better recognise the paradoxical, ambivalent, daimonic nature of illness we can learn to interact with it more fully. We will respond intelligently with more than the mind alone and we will respond with more than an arsenal of weapons and techniques. Our main aim will not necessarily be to create distance and objectivity. Instead we will aim to enlist the intelligence of the heart, body, and soul. We will engage instinct, sensitivity, feeling, humour, and poise. We have noted how these elements of healing were refined and incorporated into the approach of the ancient healers in the Greek Asklepieia.

Chöd

Let us look at how we might approach illness in this more accepting and positive way. Once again we can find inspiration and learn from Eastern cultures. Take for example the Tibetan Buddhist spiritual practice known as Chöd (pronounced "chuhd"). It is believed to have originated and been developed in the eleventh and twelfth centuries by a female teacher or "yogini" by the name of Machig Labdrön. It is purportedly able to deal effectively with "eighty thousand kinds of obstructing forces" and "404 kinds of disease" (Harding, 2003, p. 110). It is said of its practitioners "that they become immune to infectious diseases" (Allione, 2008, p. 119). At times of outbreak of smallpox or cholera its practitioners were reportedly called upon to care for the afflicted and to help deal with the bodies of the dead. It was believed that they themselves would not be affected (Allione, 2008, p. 119).

The method involves making a counterintuitive response to the illness. Instead of fighting the condition, the practitioner actively offers him or herself to it. By giving energy or "feeding" the disease with the attention it demands, the "demon" of the disease is believed to loosen its hold. Here we can see a very clear analogy with the process of psychotherapy. As psychotherapists we tend to think less in terms of "demons". We generally prefer to think more in terms of attending with interest to the underlying psychological significance of the energy carried by the pathology and its symptoms. We do this with the aim of enabling the client or sufferer to meet the needs and demands of the illness in a more conscious way. In this way we hope to foster greater wholeness and health.

Chöd practitioner Tsultrim Allione recounts the story of a friend of hers who suffered with auto immune deficiency syndrome (AIDS). The count of his "helper T cells" had fallen to a dangerously low level and was continuing to drop. He was participating in a clinical study which compared the effectiveness of azidothymidine (AZT—a drug used to delay the development of AIDS) with a placebo remedy. He did not know which treatment group he was a part of. He had seen many of his friends die slowly and horribly of the condition and felt that his fear was the worst part of his illness.

Allione encouraged him to face his fear head-on by visualising his illness as a demon and asking what it wanted of him. He pictured it in the form of a monstrous parasitic green amoeba. The illness said it wanted to take his life slowly and to see him grow "thin, sick, and weak" until he was "debilitated and ugly" and then finally to watch him die. The demon seemed to take a sadistic glee in his fear. It seemed to crave the power it felt in being able to make him suffer in this way.

He was given a meditation practice in which he visualised giving the demon exactly what it said that it wanted. He did this in a regular meditation practice in which he would imagine that he surrendered himself to the demon. He would relinquish in succession his blood, skin, eyesight, hair, mind, etc. By meditating in this way he said that he came to develop a "luminous-emptiness awareness" in which he lost his fear. The energy that had gone into his fear now went into his spiritual practice. After completing his clinical treatment and while persisting with the meditation, he learned that he had been in the placebo group during the medical trial. Despite this his T cell count had climbed back into the normal range where it continued to remain over many years (2008, pp. 120–124).

Yakun Natima

Let us take a look at another even more ancient approach to healing which is believed to have been contemporary with the Greek Asklepieia while yet it still lives on today. As we understand was the case in Greece, it too has worked since ancient times side by side with methodologies based on rational observation. However, unlike what had been the case in Greece, its spiritual, intuitive, and artistic traditions have survived the millennia. The probable last vestiges of this dying custom are performed today on the Indian Ocean island of Sri Lanka. It is known locally as the "Yakun Natima" or the "devil dance ritual". It dramatically enacts in a concrete way many of the concepts we have been exploring.

Visitors to the island will be familiar with a local tradition of making grotesque masks often with distorted faces, bulging eyes, and fangs. These are meant to represent illnesses and are widely available as souvenirs. They derive from a ceremony which is performed in villages in the southern part of the island. It is offered to people who are considered to be "possessed" by a "yakka" or the demon of an illness. As is the case with Chöd, the illness is seen as an entity that has a purpose and a personality. It is considered to be possible to enter into dialogue with it and to reach an appeasement. In an elaborate night time ceremony the demon of the illness is conjured up in a ritual. In the course of the ceremony a grotesquely masked dancer is considered to become an embodiment of the demon of the illness so that a dialogue can occur.

> They acknowledge the influence and power of the yakka as both the cause and the cure. They recite their histories, extol their power, and pay tribute to their prowess. These ceremonies are designed to call forth the "essence" of the offending demon. Through sweet-talk

and offerings or through cajoling and threats, the yakka is made to remove the affliction. (Pate, 2014)

The ceremony takes place over the course of a whole night. Darkness is conducive to finding the emotional and daimonic aspects of illness; rather than then the bright light of day which favours clarity, distance, and rational thought. It is sometimes performed in the patient's home with the extended family present or otherwise fully in public with the whole village present in addition to anyone else who wishes to attend. As we've discussed, illness can be seen as more than personal. It is a matter of relevance and concern to the family and the community. The ritual acknowledges that illness has its roots both in the social and spiritual dimensions.

The ceremony is prepared by first making offerings to the "ghosts" usually of dead kin. In our terms we could liken this to the inherited patterns of behaviour or to family and social patterns that a sufferer may have unconsciously adopted. These might be pathogenic and maladapted to present conditions and liable to undermine the authentic self and the patient's life's purpose. The offerings are made in little baskets which are meant to contain the ghosts for the duration of the ceremony. The offerings are usually of food, alcohol, tobacco, or sometimes of other delicacies such as marijuana and opium thought likely to appeal to the ghosts that induce illness (Kapferer, 1983, p. 190). In psychotherapy we also aim to acknowledge and name the familial influences from the past that underpin our issues. We do this in order that we might hand back to their rightful owners issues that are not intrinsically our own.

Numerous rituals are then performed to cleanse the ceremonial space and to summon up helpful spirits. Particular tribute is paid to the Buddha to whom it is believed that all illnesses are ultimately subservient. Here again as psychotherapists we can recognise the need for a contained space, for safe boundaries within which the work of therapy can be done. We too need to be mindful of our guiding principles and inspiring figures in the work of attending to soul. The "Buddha" simply refers to the "awakened one". Buddhism is regarded as no more and no less than the process of becoming fully awakened. All illnesses are considered to be subordinate to the power of this awakening. Psychotherapy shares the goal of the healing through wakefulness. Most of us hold that bringing unconscious issues to consciousness enables life to be lived without the neurotic misery to which Freud referred.

The ceremony itself is a complex matter that involves prayers, chanting, drumming, poetry recitation, and the telling of myths and legends which contextualise the sufferings of the patient. These are intended to evoke both the demons of disease as well as powers of healing. Songs are sung that are meant to induce emotional states in the patient that are regarded as helpful to the healing ritual. We can see an analogy with the healing approach of the Asklepieia where the arts were used to create a cathartic environment where subliminal and withheld emotions could be acknowledged and released. Many forms of psychotherapy also recognise the value and importance of catharsis in the healing process.

The exorcist (who is always a man in this tradition) offers his own body to the disease entity. It is supposed that because he is immune from affliction by the malady he is therefore better equipped than the patient to deal with it. Perhaps as psychotherapists we do something analogous in giving ourselves to the therapy process. Our capacity and aspiration is to offer unconditional empathy and full presence to the client. While we endeavour not take on board the client's issues as though they were our own, we do offer our fullest support in the expectation that it will strengthen the client's capacity to face and to manage their issues.

The night proceeds with a great variety of rituals, songs, and dances. Some of these are meant to shock and to terrify the patient in order to "jolt the patient (so) that the demon's grip on the patient is loosened" (Kapferer, 1983, p. 210). While this is not something we would aim to do in the course of psychotherapy, it is however reminiscent of the psychiatric technique of electro convulsive therapy or ECT which is intended to jolt people out of severe depression and other mental states.

Other dances and songs are intended to be comic, crude, lavatorial, and sexual. Again as in the Asklepieia primal energies are awakened and stirred both in the patient and amongst the attendees of the audience. The beneficial power of laughter is invited to become a part of the healing process. Humour, so long as it is not dismissive, belittling, or avoidant, can also be an important part of effective psychotherapy. The healing power of humour is well attested by the American journalist Norman Cousins who tells of a time when he fell ill and was medically diagnosed to have a painful, debilitating, and life threatening illness called "ankylosing spondylitis". This is an incurable spinal column disease of unknown cause.

His doctor told him that he had a one in five hundred chance of a full recovery and added that he personally had never known of anyone who had recovered from the condition (1979, p. 33). Cousins felt little confidence in his hospital treatment. He therefore felt inclined to ignore the advice of his doctors. He prescribed himself mega doses of vitamin C and he reasoned that as his condition had come to a head at a time of stress he would aim to relax. He arranged to leave the hospital, rent a hotel room, and hire a nurse to attend to him. In order to counteract his stress he spent a month doing what he enjoyed most; namely watching humorous films and television shows, reading comic books, and writing jokes. He found that the more he was able to find relief in laughter the better he was able to sleep without pain.

After a month of this self-prescribed treatment he returned to the hospital for a check-up. He was then told that he no longer had any trace of his disease. He abandoned his medication after two weeks and was able to return to work after six months. He died sixteen years later at the age of seventy-five.

Cousins had rediscovered the "best of all medicines"; the restorative power of humour and laughter. The highly influential seventeenth century English physician Thomas Sydenham declared that "the arrival of a good clown exercises a more beneficial influence upon the health of a town than of twenty asses laden with drugs" (Burch, 2010, p. 31). This knowledge has been well known and put to good use since the most ancient of times as we have noted with regard to the Asklepieia and in the case of the Yakun Natima ceremony that we are presently describing.

Powerful protective spiritual forces are summoned up in the ritual and a number of empty chairs are placed in front of the patient. What follows, we as psychotherapists might well regard as the ultimate in "empty chair work". Upon these chairs are placed a succession of "offerings baskets". These contain food and other gifts considered to be attractive to the demons of illness. To the rhythm of drumbeats the demons are summoned up one by one. As their stories are told they duly appear in the form of threateningly masked dancers who are considered to be possessed by the spirits of the illness. In the main they behave atrociously as one might expect from demons. They spit, they fart, and they belch. They make crude sexual remarks. They lurch forward and sprout fangs and they make violent threats, but they also enter into a dialogue with the exorcist. The ritual, taking place as it does in the dead of night, creates a mesmerising trancelike atmosphere through this bizarre mix of comedy, fear, mythology, and spirituality. It has the effect of taking the patient beyond the confines of the illness solely as it manifests in their own psyche and body. The patient and the illness become part of a greater drama enacted on both the earthly and spiritual planes. It contextualises the sufferings of the patient both into a community of supernatural forces and into the human community of the spectators and participants in the ritual.

This interchange with and confrontation of the demons is considered to restore a cosmic order. Through the recitation of myths and mantras, the singing of songs, recitation of poems, the performing of dance and drama, along with the evocation of higher spiritual powers, the demons are reminded of their relatively lowly place in the hierarchy of the cosmos. They are obliged by the exorcist and the powers he evokes to relinquish their hold upon the patient and remove the disease.

Rachel

Psychotherapists are of course not exorcists. Or, is there perhaps a sense in which they are? Certainly Rollo May reckoned that it is "the task of the therapist [...] to conjure up the devils, rather than put them to sleep" (1970, p. 201). Sometimes in the course of therapy it may be helpful to visualise the illness in order to better understand its nature and what it demands of us. Sometimes too when we are in the grip of a physical or psychological illness we could, figuratively speaking, imagine this as a kind of "possession". On some occasions this analogy is hard to ignore. Such was the case with Rachel, a young Israeli woman on a year's work placement in the UK who was seeking psychotherapy.

She explained that she had come to therapy because she was afraid she would lose her friends due to her behaviour when she got drunk. She had been in the UK for only three months and now found that after a few drinks she would flare up into uncontrollable tempers. She had no memory of what she did but her friends told her that she would "speak in tongues", grunt and groan like an animal, and gnash her teeth. Sometimes her friends could scarcely hold her back from attacking strangers in the street. When asked about how she normally dealt with her anger she replied that she was "never angry". Far from it, she was in fact the "family peacemaker". She went on to explain that this had been the case at least since the age of five. At that time she had witnessed her father in a drunken rage attempting to kill her mother by suffocating her with a cushion. She believed that it was only because of her protests that her mother had survived.

Shortly after this her parents divorced. She gradually lost contact with her father. He was only ever spoken about by her mother in terms of his being a "devil" or an "animal". She said that she had hated her father all her life. However, since coming to the UK she said that she was surprised to find that her feelings about him had become more intense. She found herself preoccupied with compulsive recurring hateful thoughts about him. She was puzzled by this because when she heard that he had died three years earlier she "couldn't have cared less".

Early in her therapy she dreamed that she:

> [...] is aboard a tram in her home city when another tram passes from the opposite direction. A hand reaches out of the window of the oncoming tram and offers her a bag of sweets which she accepts. A person beside her tells her that she should give them back.

This reminded her of the time when her parents were still together. It was a time before she had learned to hate her father and he would bring her sweets. Later on she would reject his sweets. She cried deeply as she recounted this. She recalled that her father had friends who thought that he was a good man. He had in fact once won an award for bravery when he risked his life by moving a terrorist bomb to a safe place in his truck. The dream raised the possibility that she might have some positive feelings about her father.

She began to explore her forgotten feelings of anger and rage at her father and at how this impacted on her present relationship. At night she sometimes began to lie awake having fantasies about her father. On one occasion she imagined addressing him as "Dad" and felt shocked that such a familiar and friendly word had occurred to her. On another occasion she imagined meeting him on the opposite side of a table that was floating in the sea. She didn't speak to him and he didn't look at her but she regarded this as the first time she'd ever confronted him even in fantasy. She said she put the table in the sea because she didn't know if he belonged in heaven or in hell.

As she opened up to the possibility that her father might not be all bad, she was more able to separate her capacity for self-assertion from her anger and rage. She became less of a peacemaker and found that she was able to deal effectively with a friend by whom she felt bullied.

She became more aware of the issues that underpinned her state of apparent "possession". She reported one week that she had again got drunk. When she was in this state her boyfriend had unjustly accused her of infidelity. She flew into a rage and attacked him with a knife. Even as she raised the knife to strike him she realised that it was not him but her father that she wanted to kill. She then turned the knife against herself and attempted to slash her own wrist. Her boyfriend managed to restrain her but she bit deeply into his hand. He called the police for assistance but by the time they arrived she had calmed down.

She was able in therapy to review the incident and to make a clear distinction between her feelings about her boyfriend and those relating to her father. She understood that she habitually dealt with her boyfriend and with men in general with a pre-emptive strike. She wanted to hurt them before they had a chance to hurt her.

Rachel returned to Israel for a short stay with the intention of visiting her father's grave in the company of a friend of hers who she thought would be supportive. She wanted to deal more deeply with her feelings about him. Her main fear was that her mother might reject her if she knew that she was trying to reconsider the role of her father in her life.

Upon her return to the UK she said that she had not yet found the courage to visit the grave of her father but that she had had a long talk with her mother. For the first time her mother was prepared to open up. She could now see that her mother also had an angry side. She could see that her father was "just human" and neither a devil nor an animal. She felt reassured that her mother cared deeply for her and much more grounded because her earliest memories were now validated by someone else. After these experiences she ended the relationship she was in. She became able to keep her drinking under control and said she had no problems with violent feelings. She was no longer subject to her states of apparent "possession".

Rollo May says that:

> The one way to get over daimonic possession is to possess it, by frankly confronting it, coming to terms with it, integrating it into the self-system. (1970, p. 201)

The irrational feelings expressed during her states of possession had now become more conscious. She had successfully begun to contextualise these feelings within the dynamics of her family, her relationship, and her social circle. She had begun to confront the "ghosts" of her past. Her pathology had lessened and she was more able to direct her energy in ways that improved her circumstances. She had found the light hidden within the darkness, the angel behind the demon. She had discovered the gift of self-awareness hidden within her fiendish violent drunken outbursts. What had manifested as a devil, a vicious animal, or a demon proved to have a health giving and life enhancing side to its nature.

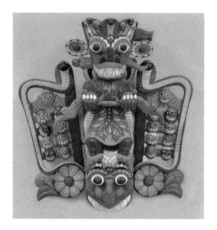

Sri Lankan Mask of Maha Kola (the Prince of illness-causing demons). The eighteen smaller masks represent his consort of lesser illness-causing demons.

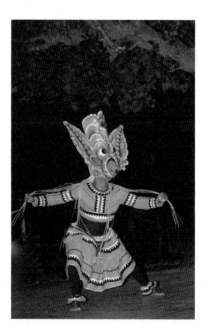

A Sri Lankan "demon dancer" believed to be "possessed" by the spirit of an illness.

CHAPTER ELEVEN

In conclusion

The mystery of life is not a problem to be solved; it is a reality to be experienced.

—*Jacobus Johannes Leeuw* (1928, p. 9)

Readers from the psychotherapy world who came to this volume in the hope or expectation of adding further tools to their psychotherapeutic "tool kits" will in all probability have succumbed to disappointment and/or annoyance long before reaching this concluding chapter. It will be obvious by now that this is neither a "fix it" manual to help to mend a broken psyche nor is it a cookbook of recipes to enliven psychotherapy sessions that have become dull and predictable. After all who is it that would be doing the repairs or cooking up the latest offering? What is the psychology of that person? To what values and priorities does the fixer adhere? What assumptions does he or she hold?

Can we learn to skilfully manipulate the psyche to provide us with the happiness, peace, contentment, and fulfilment that we desire? Can we live in the light without darkness or would we then become snow blind and unable to see anything at all. Is it really so much more desirable to be blinded by the light than it is to be lost in the darkness? In neither case can we find our way.

What we have preferred to dwell on here is the unfathomable, paradoxical, ambivalent, and daimonic; those qualities that relativise the ego and stifle it in its quest to take charge and run the show. The ego is a part of the psyche. The psyche is the greater force. Jung says that we are like fish in the ocean of the psyche. Bearing in mind that not everyone sees things in this way he speculates that "perhaps there are also fishes who believe they contain the sea" (1931a, p. 180).

But surely people come to therapy because they want solutions to problems and answers to questions. That's what they pay for. Yes indeed and that's also probably a large part of the reason why they're "dis-eased". It is the desire for control and the fear of surrender and letting go that blocks the flow of life. If we address problems within the terms in which we have defined them we limit the scope of new energies to enter our lives. Such blocked energy is prone to manifest in ways that are pathological. We become susceptible to dissociated states among which are psychological and physical illnesses. And yes psychological theory can offer an enlarged framework within which a client may reframe their concerns and find resolution to certain of their conflicts. However, the healing or wholing is not an intellectual exercise. It does not come primarily from theory. It comes from a person's willingness and capacity to risk opening up and stepping into the unknown.

A psychotherapist who offers solutions to problems and answers to questions is not a psychotherapist in the etymological sense of being a soul attendant. Such a psychotherapist risks disempowering the client and disconnecting them from their own capacity to find their way in life. The psychotherapist is not a problem solver or heroic rescuer. Answers to questions are likely to shut the psyche down. Having found the answer we may no longer find it necessary to dwell on the self-discovery that occurs when confused emerging emotions arise. Answers tend to conclude matters. Questions on the other hand offer us ways forward and possible new directions.

So without answers and without solutions the work of psychotherapy, or attending to the soul, can at times be pretty nerve wracking. We may be confronted with a suffering client anxiously and hopefully expecting a service we do not provide. It is then that we must practice the supreme art of what psychotherapist Thomas Moore calls "sitting on a chair without wobbling".

> I don't think it is my job to do anything to the person—not teach
> him, not cure him, not make him healthy, not even help him. Of
> course, one's intention is always to help, but I believe that if I have
> the specific intention of helping, our work will be ruined from the
> start. (1996, p. 181)

So if we are not there to support the ego in its quest to regain its grip
on the direction of life and the mastery and eradication of its symptoms
what is the alternative? We have put forward the idea that the alternative is "to attend to the soul", to put ourselves in the service of that
greater entity of which the ego is a component part. We don't do this
primarily with a set of therapeutic techniques. We do this instead with
the fullest presence that we are able to summons.

Whilst keeping our best attention on the client we see, hear, feel, and
intuit what they communicate to us both consciously and deliberately
and unconsciously. We aim to remain present in the fullest awareness
of which we are capable. We remain un-swayed by judgements either
of the client or of ourselves. As Thomas Moore might say we do not
"wobble".

We try to provide an atmosphere in which psyche's voice can be
heard, trusting that forces greater than either ourselves or the client
will further the process of healing. We have "faith" in this force or process. Alexander Lowen, the originator of bioenergetic psychotherapy
explains what he understands by this kind of faith.

> Letting go of ego control means giving in to the body in its invol-
> untary aspect. It means letting the body take over. But this is what
> patients cannot do. *They feel the body will betray them.* They do not
> trust it and have no faith in it. They are afraid that if the body takes
> over, it will expose their weakness, demolish their pretentiousness,
> reveal their sadness, and vent their fury. Yes, it will do that. It will
> destroy the facades that people erect to hide their true selves from
> themselves and from the world. But it will also open a new depth
> of being and add a richness to life compared to which the wealth of
> the world is a mere trifle. (1972, p. 305)

"True faith" Lowen asserts, "is a commitment to the life of the spirit—
the spirit that resides in the body of a person" (1972, p. 214). This
"spirit" that is manifest in the "body" is what we have preferred to call

the daimonic. It is not something that can be pinned down. It cannot be known except as Jung says through the power of the imagination, the "imaginal", or our inborn aptitude to form images.

As psychotherapists we are therefore interested in the language of the psyche; the metaphors, symbols, and symptoms that arise in the course of the work. The more compelling these are the more attentively we listen. We suspect that the energetic charge carried by an impressive and often troubling image or symptom may also carry with it the potential for a meaningful and creative transformation. We know from psychoneuroimmunoendocrinology (PNI) and placebo research studies that scientific medicine is just beginning to appreciate the immense healing potential of the imagination. We are learning that the spiritual origins of our own medical tradition and the exotic spiritual healing methods of some cultures distant from us cannot be lightly dismissed. It is clear that these are not simply primitive superstitions clung to by those who have yet to discover the benefits of a scientific approach to healing.

We realise that our role as psychotherapists who work directly with the imagination is central to the healing process. Our work is not merely an adjunct to be employed when conditions are regarded as "only" psychological. We have evidence that our work is more than this and we know it from our own experience. When clients get to the root of their psychological issues the state of their physical health can also respond in sometimes dramatic and remarkable ways. When a client is able to uncover and release the energy held within a symptom it leads to greater wholeness or health. The result can be relief from symptoms and improved wellbeing.

To get to this point we must endure the paradoxical predicament of accepting and even valuing the very condition that has brought us into therapy in the hope of finding relief. We must accept the symptoms and illness which we wish to reject. And conversely we must reject our desire to be rid of them. In 2003 a Swedish company developed a game called "Mindball". It is a two person game in which players compete to roll a ball across a table toward their opponent using only the power of their brainwaves. These are monitored by a headset which controls the movement of the ball. Brain rhythms indicative of deep relaxation propel the ball forward toward the opponent. The competitor who is most relaxed and, in effect, the least competitive wins the competition.

An active desire to win ensures a loss while the ability to accept and to deal with loss optimises the likelihood of winning. Such can also be the paradox of healing.

In the Chinese Taoist philosophy this approach is known as "wu wei" or "not doing". Not doing should not however be understood to be a state of passivity, disengagement, and resignation. It is far from being this. It is a state of relaxed conscious acceptance of what is. It is a kind of faith or trust in life. It is a confidence that life is taking us where we must necessarily go. We find our strength not so much in our ability to redirect life in ways that are pleasing to the ego, but in our capacity to value the experience we are actually having. As Lowen indicated, our strength lies more in our ability to live skilfully and creatively accepting ourselves just as we discover ourselves to be. The greatest personal change that we can make as individuals is not to transform ourselves into the ego's ideal of who we would like to become. It is to accept ourselves as we truly are. The paradox is that we change most profoundly by ceasing to try to change ourselves. The deepest psychological change is a matter of "homecoming", self-realisation, self-actualisation, or individuation. We become the person we have always been but have never before fully dis-covered or re-membered. We have, as James Hillman says, "grown down". We have done the work of what we have called the "personal daimon" and become manifest in the world as the person we are meant to be. When we bring this person into the world we become at last fully born and present. The role of the psychotherapist is in this sense to be a kind of midwife to the soul.

We have stressed that to best enable this process to happen we need to overcome our tendency to create psychological tension by thinking in terms of opposites. The more we strive for predetermined goals and outcomes the greater will be the temptation to reject and suppress that which blocks our way. In this way we energise the opposites that we need to get beyond. We tend to want light but not darkness, health but not illness, harmony but not conflict, joy but not sorrow, etc. We must look below or behind these opposites. We must take the deeper view that is demanded of us by the psyche. The psyche delivers to us both our joys and our woes. It engenders our illnesses and symptoms as it strives for realisation. The Lebanese artist, poet, and writer Kahlil Gibran put it this way.

The deeper that sorrow carves into your being, the more joy you can contain.

When you are joyous, look deep into your heart and you shall find it is only that which has given you sorrow that is giving you joy. (1926, p. 36)

William Blake put it this way.

> Man was made for Joy & Woe
> And when this we rightly know
> Thro' the World we safely go,
> Joy and woe are woven fine,
> A Clothing for the Soul divine;
> Under every grief & pine
> Runs a joy with silken twine. (1946, pp. 151–152)

As psychotherapeutic soul attendants we put our faith in the flow of life. We could call this flow the Tao which literally means "the path" or "the way." It is not subject to the control of either therapist or client. In the Western world we learn from the Anglo Saxon tradition in the epic poem Beowolf, which is believed to have been written sometime between the eighth to eleventh centuries, that "fate ever goes as fate must" (Heaney, 2009, line 455) This principle of the inexorability of fate was known in old English as the "wyrd". According to the psychologist and writer Brian Bates the wyrd was regarded as a "creative, organic vision paralleling the classical Eastern concept of Yin and Yang" (1996, p. 6). It imagined the cosmos as an interconnected three dimensional web in which "any event anywhere, resulted in reverberations and repercussions throughout the web". In order to live skilfully and fully it was considered necessary to be present to and aware of this infinitely greater vision. While in ancient Greece we have noted that it was the daughter of the goddess Ananke or "Necessity" who was believed to put before us our life choices. It was Necessity who required her to allocate to us our personal daimon; the daimon whose job it is to remind us of our purpose in life. The paradox of health is that we must learn to live in willing accord with that which Necessity demands of us. We must become the people we truly are and fully inhabit the life that we actually lead.

REFERENCES

Abram, D. (1996). *The Spell of the Sensuous: Perception and Language in a More-Than-Human World*. New York: Vintage.

Abram, D. (2010). *Becoming Animal: An Earthly Cosmology*. New York: Pantheon.

Agius, M. (2008). A dissenting voice. *New Therapist 55*: 22.

Al Ghazali, A. H. (1909). *The Alchemy of Happiness*, New York: Cosimo Classics.

Allione, T. (2008). *Feeding your Demons: Ancient Wisdom for Resolving Inner Conflict*. London: Hay House.

Amanzio, M., Latini, L., Vase, C.L., & Benedetti, F. (2009). A systemic review of adverse events in placebo groups of anti-migraine clinical trials. *Pain 146(3)*: 261–269.

Bates, B. (1996). *The Wisdom of the Wyrd: Teachings for Today from our Ancient Past*, London: Rider & Co.

Bates, K. L. (2008). You get what you pay for? Costly placebo works better than cheap one. *Duke Today, Mar 5*.

Bertini, I. (2014). London's Oxford street has 'world's highest' levels of diesel fumes. *Blue & Green Tomorrow Online Newsletter, 6 Jul*.

Bible (1946). *The Holy Bible; The New Testament*. New York: Collins.

Bible (1970). *The New English Bible*. Oxford: Oxford & Cambridge Press.

Blake, W. (1946). *The Essential Blake*. London: Chatto & Windus.

Bleakley, A. (1984). *Fruits of the Moontree: The Medicine Wheel & Transpersonal Psychology*. Bath, UK: Gateway.

Bolte-Taylor, J. (2008). *My Stroke of Insight*. London: Hodder.

Bosnak, R. (2007). *Embodiment; Creative Imagination in Medicine, Art and Travel*. London: Routledge.

Bottrell, W. (1873). *Traditions and Hearthside Stories of West Cornwall, Second Series*. Lampeter, UK: Llanerch.

Burch, D. (2010). *Taking the Medicine: A Short History of Medicine's Beautiful Idea, and Our Difficulty in Swallowing It*. London: Vintage.

Calaprice, A. (1950). *The New Quotable Einstein*. Princeton, NJ: Princeton University Press.

Cameron, D. (2010). Placebos work—even without deception. *Harvard Gazette, 22 Dec.*

Chalquist, C. (2007). *Terrapsychology: Reengaging the Soul of Place*. New Orleans: Spring.

Chatwin, B. (1987). *The Songlines*. Harmondsworth: Penguin.

Conger, J. (1994). *The Body in Recovery: Somatic Psychotherapy and the Self*. Berkeley, CA: Frog Books.

Cowan, J. C. (1992). *The Elements of the Aboriginal Tradition*. Shaftsbury, UK: Element.

Cousins, N. (1979). *Anatomy of an Illness as Perceived by the Patient: Reflections on Healing and Regeneration*. London: Norton.

Dangerous Laboratories (2014). *Trenwith Mine: St. Ives*. Dangerous Laboratories. Available at: www.dangerouslaboratories.org/rcw6.html. Retrieved 30/10/14

Dach, J. (2014). *Natural Solutions with Bio Identical Hormones*. Available at: www.drdach.com/wst_page8.html. Retrieved 16/7/14.

Dennis, S. L. (2001). *Embrace of the Daimon: Healing through the Subtle Energy Body/Jungian Psychology & the Dark Feminine*. York Beach, ME: Nicolas-Hayes.

Dethlefesen, T. & Dahlke, R. (1991). *The Healing Power of Illness: Understanding What Your Symptoms are Telling You*. Shaftsbury, UK: Element.

Duff, K. (1993). *The Alchemy of Illness*. New York: Bell Tower.

Edelstein, E. J., & Edelstein, L. (1945). *Asclepius: Collection and Interpretation of the Testimonies*. Baltimore: Johns Hopkins.

Eliade, M. (1964). *Shamanism: Archaic Techniques of Ecstasy*. London: Arkana.

Eyesenck, H. J. (1952). The Effects of Psychotherapy: An Evaluation, *Journal of Consulting Psychology, Vol. 16(5)*: 319–324.

Ferris, D. (2014). Godrevey and Gwithian community demonstration against sewage pollution. *Surfers Against Sewage, Jul 22*. Available at: www.sas.org.uk/news/campaigns/godrevy-gwithian-community-demonstration-against-sewage-pollution/. Retrieved 16/8/14.

Freud, S. & Breuer, J. (1895d). *Studies on Hysteria. S.E. 2*. London: Hogarth.

Freud, S. (1900a). *The Interpretation of Dreams. S.E. 4 & 5*. London: Hogarth.

Freud, S. In: L. Andreas-Salomé (1965). *The Freud Journal*. London: Hogarth.

Friedlander, W. J. (1992). *The Golden Wand of Medicine: A History of the Caduceus Symbol in Medicine*. New York: Greenwood Press.

Gibran, K. (1926). *The Prophet*. London: Heinemann.

Goldacre, B. (2012). *Bad Pharma: How drug companies mislead doctors and harm patients*. London: Harper Collins.

Graves, R. (1959). *Larousse Encyclopedia of Mythology*. London: Paul Hamlyn.

Greenson, R. R. (1967). *The Technique and Practice of Psycho-Analysis: The International Psycho-Analytical Library 74*. London: Hogarth Press and Institute of Psycho-Analysis.

Groddeck, G. (1923). *The Book of the It*. London: Vision.

Groddeck, G. (1970). *The Meaning of Illness: Selected Psychoanalytic Writings*. Madison, CT: International Universities Press.

Hahn T. N. (1988). *The Heart of Understanding: Commentaries on the Prajnaparamita Heart Sutra*. Berkeley, CA: Parallax.

Hahn T. N. (1993). *The Blooming of a Lotus: Guided Meditation Exercises for Healing and Transformation*. Boston, MA: Beacon.

Harding, S. (2003). *Machik's Complete Explanation: Clarifying the Meaning of Chöd*. Ithaca, NY: Snow Lion.

Harpur, P. (1994). *Daimonic Reality: A Field Guide to the Otherworld*. London: Viking Arkana.

Hart, G. D. (2000). *Asclepius the God of Medicine*. London: Royal Society of Medicine.

Heaney, S. (2009). *Beowolf*. London: Faber & Faber.

Hegde, B. M. (2006). *What Doctors Don't Get to Study in Medical School*. Tunbridge Wells, UK: Anshan.

Hillman, J. (1975). *Re-visioning Psychology*. London: HarperCollins.

Hillman, J. (2000). *Pan and the Nightmare*. Woodstock, CT: Spring Publications.

Hillman, J., & Ventura, M. (1992). *We've Had a Hundred Years of Psychotherapy and the World's Getting Worse*. San Francisco: HarperCollins.

Holmes, R. (1974). *Witchcraft in History*. Secaucus, NJ: Citadel Press.

Homer (1969), *Iliad*. Harmondsworth: Penguin.

Houston, J. (1987). *The Search for the Beloved: Journeys in Mythology and Sacred Psychology*. Los Angeles: Tarcher.

Huber, M. (2011). Health—How should we define it? *British Medical Journal, 26 Jul. 343*. Published online doi: 10.1136/bmj.d4163. Retrieved 14/8/15.

Hughs, D. A. (2011). Report endorses German GP's use of placebos, *The Guardian, 6 Mar.*

Illich, I. (1976). *Limits to Medicine: Medical Nemesis—The Expropriation of Health*. Harmondsworth: Pelican.

Jeanty, J. (2014). *Lithium and Liver Function*. Available at: www.ehow.com/ about_6362060_lithium-liver-function.html. Retrieved 14/8/15.

Jung, C. G. (1921). *Psychological Types, Collected Works, Volume 6*. London: Routledge & Kegan Paul.

Jung, C. G. (1931a). Commentary. In: R. Wilhelm (Trans.) *The Secret of the Golden Flower: A Chinese Book of Life*. New York: Harvest.

Jung, C. G. (1931b). *The Structure and Dynamics of the Psyche (2nd edn), Collected Works, Volume 8*. London: Routledge & Kegan Paul.

Jung, C. G. (1933). *Modern Man in Search of a Soul*. London: Routledge.

Jung, C. G. (1935). In: J. L. Jarret (1997). *Jung's Seminar on Nietzsche's Zarathustra*. Princeton, NJ: Bollingen Series XCIX.

Jung, C. G. (1941). *The Practice of Psychotherapy, Collected Works (2nd edn), Volume 16*. London: Routledge & Kegan Paul.

Jung, C. G. (1956). *Symbols of Transformation (2nd edn), Collected Works, Volume 5*, London: Routledge & Kegan Paul.

Jung, C. G. (1958). *Psychology and Religion West and East (2nd edn), Collected Works, Volume 11*. London: Routledge & Kegan Paul.

Jung, C. G. (1961). *Memories, Dreams, Reflections*, London: Collins and Routledge.

Jung, C. G. (1964). *Civilisation in Transition (2nd edn), Collected Works, Volume 10*. London: Routledge & Kegan Paul.

Jung, C. G. (2002). *The Earth has a Soul: the Nature Writings of C. G. Jung*. Sabini, M. (Ed.). Berkeley, CA: North Atlantic.

Kapferer, B. (1983). A *Celebration of Demons: Exorcism and the Aesthetics of Healing in Sri Lanka*. Washington DC: Smithsonian Institute.

Kaptchuk, T., & Croucher, M. (1986). *The Healing Arts: Exploring the Medical Ways of the World*. London: British Broadcasting Corporation.

Kerényi, C. (1959). *Asklepios: Archetypal Image of the Physician's Existence*. London: Thames & Hudson.

King, H. (2001). *Greek and Roman Medicine*. Bristol: Bristol Classical.

Kirsch, I, Deacon, B. J., Huedo-Medina, T. B., Scoboria, A., Moore, T. J., & Johnson, B. T. (2008). Initial severity and antidepressant benefits: A meta-analysis of data submitted to the food and drug administration. *New Therapist, 55*: 11–21.

Kitman, J. (2000). *The secret history of lead. The Nation, 20 Mar.*

Kreinheder, A. (1991). *Body and Soul: The Other Side of Illness*. Toronto: Inner City Books.

Laing, R. D. (1961). *Self and Others*. Harmondsworth: Pelican.

Laing, R. D. (1967). *The Politics of Experience and The Bird of Paradise*. Harmondsworth: Penguin.

Leeuw, J. J. (1928). *The Conquest of Illusion*. London: Knopf.

Lehrer, J. (2010). Depression's upside. *New York Times Sunday Magazine* *28 Feb. MM38.*

Liccardi, G., et al. (2004). Evaluation of the nocebo effect during oral challenge in patients with adverse drug reactions. *Journal of Investigational Allergology and Clinical Immunology No. 14(2)*: 104–107. Retrieved 14/8/15.

Linde, C., Gadler, F., Kappenberger, L., & Rydén, L. (1999). Placebo effect of pacemaker implantation in obstructive hypertrophis cardiomyopathy. *American Journal of Cardiology, March 15, 83(6)*: 903–907. Retrieved 14/8/15.

Lowen, A. (1972). *Depression and the Body: The Biological Basis of Faith and Reality.* Harmondsworth: Penguin.

Madrigal, A. C. (2011). The Dark Side of the Placebo Effect; When Intense Belief Kills. *The Atlantic Monthly, Sep 14.*

Makins, M. (Ed.) (1979). *Collins English Dictionary.* Glasgow: HarperCollins.

Maslow, A. (1968). *Toward a Psychology of Being.* New York: Van Nostrand.

Maté, G. (2003). *When the Body Says No: Exploring the Stress-Disease Connection.* Hoboken, NJ: Wiley.

May, R. (1969). *Love and Will.* London: Collins.

May, R. (1970). Psychotherapy and the daimonic. In: J. Campbell (Ed.). *Myths, Dreams and Religion.* Dallas, TX: Spring.

McGreevy, R. (2003). Drugs don't work, says Glaxo chief. *The Times, 8 Dec.*

McLees, M. N. (2000). The Tinos icon ("of great joy"). *Road to Emmaus: A Journal of Orthodox Faith and Culture, Vol 3. No 3*: 35–45.

Meade, M. (2010). *Fate and Destiny: The Two Agreements of the Soul.* Seattle: GreenFire Press.

Meador, C. (1992). Hex death: voodoo magic or persuasion? *Southern Medical Journal 85(3)*: 244–247.

Meier, C. A. (1986). *Soul and Body: Essays on the Theories of C. G. Jung.* San Francisco: Lapis Press.

Merleau-Ponty, M. (1968). *The Visible and the Invisible.* Evanston, IL: Northwestern University Press.

Miller, H. (1941). *The Colossus of Maroussi.* Harmondsworth: Penguin.

Miller, R. J. (Ed.) (1994). *The Complete Gospels: Annotated Scholars Version.* Salem, OR: Polebridge.

Mindell, A. (1985). *Working with the Dreaming Body.* London: Routledge.

Moore, T. (1990). *Dark Eros: The Imagination of Sadism.* Woodstock, CT: Spring Publications.

Moore, T. (1996). *The Re-enchantment of Everyday Life.* London: Harper Perennial.

Monbiot, G. (2013). Yes, lead poisoning could really be a cause of violent crime. *The Guardian Newspaper Jan 7*.

Moseley, J. B. et al. (2002). A controlled trial of arthroscopic surgery for osteoarthritis of the knee. *New England Journal of Medicine, 347*: 81–88.

Murchie, G. (1979). *The Seven Mysteries of Life: An Exploration of Science and Philosophy*. London: Rider Hutchinson.

Myers, D. G. (1986). *Psychology: 4th Edition*. New York: Worth.

National Health Service (2008). *NHS Direct Online Health Encyclopaedia*. Available at: www.nhsdirect.nhs.uk/articles/article.aspx?articleId=659. Retrieved 8/8/08.

Norris, R. P., & Yidumduma, H. (2014). Songlines and navigation in Wardaman and other aboriginal cultures. *Journal of Astronomical History and Heritage, Volume 17, Issue 2*: 1–15.

Onians, R. B. (1951/1988). *The Origins of European Thought: About the Body, the Mind, the Soul, the World, Time and Fate*. Cambridge: Cambridge University Press.

Osler, W. In: R. Taylor (2008). *White Coat Tales; Medicine's Heroes, Heritage and Misadventure*. New York: Springer.

Patton, K. C. (2009). Ancient Asklepieia: Institutional incubation and the hope of healing. In: S. Aizenstat & R. Bosnak (Eds.). *Imagination and Medicine: The Future of Healing in an Age of Neuroscience*. New Orleans: Spring, pp. 3–34.

Papavramidou, N., Papavramidis, T., & Demetriou, T. (2010). Ancient Greek and Greco–Roman methods in modern surgical treatment of cancer. *Annals of Surgical Oncology Mar; 17(3): 665–667*.

Partridge, E. (1958). *A Short Etymological Dictionary of Modern English*. London: Book Club Associates.

Pate, A. (2014). The yakun natima—devil dance ritual of Sri Lanka, *WWW Virtual Library—Sri Lanka*. Available at: www.lankalibrary.com/myths.html. Retrieved 9/11/14.

Perls, F. S. (1947). *Ego, Hunger and Aggression: A Revision of Freud's Theory and Method*. London: George Allen and Unwin.

Pert, C. (1997). *Molecules of Emotion: Why You Feel the Way You Feel*. London: Pocket Books.

Plato (1955). *The Republic*. Harmondsworth: Penguin.

Plutarch (1936). *Maralia—De Defectu Oraculorum (The Obsolescence of Oracles)*. Cambridge, MA: Loeb Classical Library.

Ramos, D. (2004). *The Psyche of the Body: A Jungian Approach to Psychosomatics*. London: Brunner-Routledge.

Robson-Scott, M. (2011). What if drugs don't work? *The Independent, 25 Oct*.

Rosenhan, D. L. (1973). On being sane in insane places. *Science, Vol. 179(4040)*: 250–258.

Safransky, S., London, S., & Zeiger, G. (2012). Conversations with a remarkable man: honouring the late James Hillman. *The Sun, Issue 439, July 2012*.

Sardello, R. (1995). *Love and the Soul: Creating a Future for Earth*. New York: Harper.

Sarno, J. E. (1998). *The Mindbody Prescription: Healing the Body, Healing the Pain*. New York: Grand Central Life & Style.

Schechter, D., Smith, A.P., Beck, J., Roach, J., Karim, R., & Azen, S. (2007). Outcomes of a mind-body treatment program for chronic back pain with no distinct structural pathology-a case series of patients diagnosed and treated as tension myositis syndrome". *Alternative Therapies in Health and Medicine 13 (5)*: 26–35.

Schouten, J. (1967). *The Rod and Serpent of Asklepios: Symbol of Medicine*. London: Elsevier.

Scott (2011). Why lead used to be added to gasoline. *Today I Found Out: Daily Knowledge Newsletter Nov 14*. Available at: www.todayifoundout. com/index.php/2011/11/why-lead-used-to-be-added-to-gasoline. Retrieved 14/8/15.

Seligman, M. E. P. (1995). The effectiveness of psychotherapy. *American Psychologist, Vol. 50, 12*: 965–974.

Sihvonen, R., Paavola, M., Malmivaara, A., & Järvinen, T. L. (2013). "Finnish degenerative meniscal lesion study (FIDELITY): a protocol for a randomised, placebo surgery controlled trial on the efficacy of arthroscopic partial meniscectomy for patients with degenerative meniscus injury with a novel 'RCT within-a-cohort' study design." *BMJ Open. 9 Mar 3(3)*. Published online 2013 March 9. doi: 10.1136/bmjopen-2012–002510.

Smith, M. L., & Glass, G. V. (1977). Meta-analysis of psychotherapy outcome studies. *American Psychologist No. 32 (University of Colorado)*.

Sontag, S. (1989/1991). *Illness as a Metaphor* and *AIDS and its Metaphors*. Harmondsworth: Penguin.

Sternberg, E. M. (2001). *The Balance Within: The Science Connecting Health with Emotions*. London: Palgrave.

Strupp, H. H., & Hadley, S. W. (1979). Specific versus non-specific factors in psychotherapy. *Archives of General Psychiatry No. 36(10)*.

Sydenham, T. (1848). *The Works of Thomas Sydenham, Vol. I*. London: The Sydenham Society.

US Department of Veterans Affairs (2014). *Returning Veterans with addictions*. Available at: www.psychiatrictimes.com/login?referrer=http%3

A//www.psychiatrictimes.com%2Freturning-veterans-addictions. Retrieved 15/10/14.

Walkenstein, E. (1975). *Shrunk to Fit*. London: Coventure.

Walker, B. G. (1983). *The Woman's Encyclopedia of Myths and Secrets*. San Francisco: Harper & Row.

Walton, A. (1979). *Asklepios: The Cult of the Greek God of Medicine*. Chicago Ridge, IL: Ares Publishers.

Wilde, O. (1994). *Collected Poems of Oscar Wilde (Wordsworth Poetry Library)*. Ware, UK: Wordsworth Editions.

Wenner, M. (2007). Humans carry more bacterial cells than human ones, *Scientific American, Nov 30*.

Wilkins, W. J. (1882). *Hindu Mythology: Vedic and Purānic*. New Delhi: Heritage Publishers.

Wilson, B., & Edington, G. (1981). *First Child, Second Child ... What Your Birth Order Means to You*. London: Souvenir Press.

World Health Organisation (1946). Preamble to the constitution of the World Health Organization as adopted by the International Health Conference, New York. *Official Records of the World Health Organization, no. 2.*

Yeats, W. B. (1959). *Mythologies*. London: MacMillan.

Ziegler, A. J. (1983). *Archetypal Medicine*. Woodstock CT: Spring.

* * *

Copyright information (in order of appearance)

the Creative Commons Attribution-NonCommercial-ShareAlike 2.0 Generic License. To view a copy of this license, visit http://creativecommons.org/licenses/by-nc-sa/2.0/ or send a letter to Creative Commons, PO Box 1866, Mountain View, CA 94042, USA.

6. Green man "The Sutton Benger Green Man—geograph.org.uk—1410673" by tristan forward. Licenced under CC BY-SA 2.0 via Wikimedia Commons—http://commons.wikimedia.org/wiki/File:The_Sutton_Benger_Green_Man_-_geograph.org.uk_-_1410673.jpg#/media/File:The_Sutton_Benger_Green_Man_-_geograph.org.uk_-_1410673.jpg

7. Sinhalese mask By Jorge Láscar from Australia (Daha Ata Sanniya—Raksha masks) [CC BY 2.0 (http://creativecommons.org/licenses/by/2.0)], via Wikimedia Commons.

8. Devil dancer By Jerzy Strzelecki (Own work) [GFDL (http://www.gnu.org/copyleft/fdl.html) or CC BY 3.0 (http://creativecommons.org/licenses/by/3.0)], via Wikimedia Commons.

9. Not required.

10. Not required.

INDEX